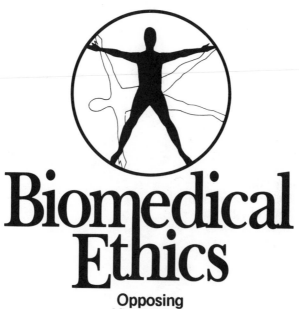

Biomedical Ethics

Opposing Viewpoints ®

Other Books of Related Interest in the Opposing Viewpoints Series:

Additional Books in the Opposing Viewpoints Series:

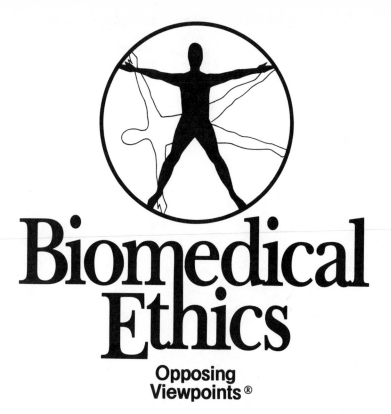

Biomedical Ethics

Opposing Viewpoints ®

David L. Bender & Bruno Leone, *Series Editors*

Julie S. Bach, *Book Editor*

Susan Bursell & Bonnie Szumski, *Assistant Editors*

OPPOSING VIEWPOINTS SERIES ®

Greenhaven Press   577 Shoreview Park Road   St. Paul, Minnesota 55126

Library of Congress Cataloging-in-Publication Data

Biomedical ethics.

(Opposing viewpoints series)
Includes bibliographies and index.
1. Medical ethics. I. Bach, Julie S., 1963-
II. Bursell, Susan, 1951-   . III. Szumski,
Bonnie, 1958-   . IV. Series.   [DNLM: 1. Bioethics.
2. Ethics, Medical.   W 50 B6156]
R724.B492   1987   174' .2   86-31921
ISBN 0-89908-396-X (lib. bdg.)
ISBN 0-89908-371-4 (pbk.)

"Congress shall make no law...
abridging the freedom of speech,
or of the press."

First Amendment to the US Constitution

The basic foundation of our democracy is the first amendment guarantee of freedom of expression. The *Opposing Viewpoints Series* is dedicated to the concept of this basic freedom and the idea that it is more important to practice it than to enshrine it.

Contents

Why Consider Opposing Viewpoints?

"It is better to debate a question without settling it than to settle a question without debating it."

Joseph Joubert (1754-1824)

The Importance of Examining Opposing Viewpoints

The purpose of the Opposing Viewpoints Series, and this book in particular, is to present balanced, and often difficult to find, opposing points of view on complex and sensitive issues.

Probably the best way to become informed is to analyze the positions of those who are regarded as experts and well studied on issues. It is important to consider every variety of opinion in an attempt to determine the truth. Opinions from the mainstream of society should be examined. But also important are opinions that are considered radical, reactionary, or minority as well as those stigmatized by some other uncomplimentary label. An important lesson of history is the eventual acceptance of many unpopular and even despised opinions. The ideas of Socrates, Jesus, and Galileo are good examples of this.

Readers will approach this book with their own opinions on the issues debated within it. However, to have a good grasp of one's own viewpoint, it is necessary to understand the arguments of those with whom one disagrees. It can be said that those who do not completely understand their adversary's point of view do not fully understand their own.

A persuasive case for considering opposing viewpoints has been presented by John Stuart Mill in his work *On Liberty*. When examining controversial issues it may be helpful to reflect on this suggestion:

> The only way in which a human being can make some approach to knowing the whole of a subject, is by hearing what can be said about it by persons of every variety of opinion, and studying all modes in which it can be looked at by every character of mind. No wise man ever acquired his wisdom in any mode but this.

Analyzing Sources of Information

The Opposing Viewpoints Series includes diverse materials taken from magazines, journals, books, and newspapers, as well as statements and position papers from a wide range of individuals, organizations and governments. This broad spectrum of sources helps to develop patterns of thinking which are open to the consideration of a variety of opinions.

Pitfalls To Avoid

A pitfall to avoid in considering opposing points of view is that of regarding one's own opinion as being common sense and the most rational stance and the point of view of others as being only opinion and naturally wrong. It may be that another's opinion is correct and one's own is in error.

Another pitfall to avoid is that of closing one's mind to the opinions of those with whom one disagrees. The best way to approach a dialogue is to make one's primary purpose that of understanding the mind and arguments of the other person and not that of enlightening him or her with one's own solutions. More can be learned by listening than speaking.

It is my hope that after reading this book the reader will have a deeper understanding of the issues debated and will appreciate the complexity of even seemingly simple issues on which good and honest people disagree. This awareness is particularly important in a democratic society such as ours where people enter into public debate to determine the common good. Those with whom one disagrees should not necessarily be regarded as enemies, but perhaps simply as people who suggest different paths to a common goal.

Developing Basic Reading and Thinking Skills

In this book, carefully edited opposing viewpoints are purposely placed back to back to create a running debate; each viewpoint is preceded by a short quotation that best expresses the author's main argument. This format instantly plunges the reader into the midst of a controversial issue and greatly aids that reader in mastering the basic skill of recognizing an author's point of view.

A number of basic skills for critical thinking are practiced in the activities that appear throughout the books in the series. Some of the skills are:

Evaluating Sources of Information The ability to choose from among alternative sources the most reliable and accurate source in relation to a given subject.

Separating Fact from Opinion The ability to make the basic distinction between factual statements (those that can be demonstrated or verified empirically) and statements of opinion (those that are beliefs or attitudes that cannot be proved).

Identifying Stereotypes The ability to identify oversimplified, exaggerated descriptions (favorable or unfavorable) about people and insulting statements about racial, religious or national groups, based upon misinformation or lack of information.

Recognizing Ethnocentrism The ability to recognize attitudes or opinions that express the view that one's own race, culture, or group is inherently superior, or those attitudes that judge another culture or group in terms of one's own.

It is important to consider opposing viewpoints and equally important to be able to critically analyze those viewpoints. The activities in this book are designed to help the reader master these thinking skills. Statements are taken from the book's viewpoints and the reader is asked to analyze them. This technique aids the reader in developing skills that not only can be applied to the viewpoints in this book, but also to situations where opinionated spokespersons comment on controversial issues. Although the activities are helpful to the solitary reader, they are most useful when the reader can benefit from the interaction of group discussion.

Using this book and others in the series should help readers develop basic reading and thinking skills. These skills should improve the reader's ability to understand what they read. Readers should be better able to separate fact from opinion, substance from rhetoric and become better consumers of information in our media-centered culture.

This volume of the Opposing Viewpoints Series does not advocate a particular point of view. Quite the contrary! The very nature of the book leaves it to the reader to formulate the opinions he or she finds most suitable. My purpose as publisher is to see that this is made possible by offering a wide range of viewpoints which are fairly presented.

David L. Bender
Publisher

Introduction

"Knowledge itself is power."

Sir Francis Bacon (1561-1626)

On a winter day in 1983, Dr. William DeVries approached a dying man and offered him one last chance at life. The man was Barney Clark. The last chance was an artificial heart called the Jarvik-7. Clark, a dentist from Seattle, faced a choice between certain, immediate death and the possibility of a few more days of life. He made the decision quickly. Most bioethical decisions, however, require longer deliberation. Conflicting views of what is right, coupled with confusion about new technology, make these choices difficult.

Before developments in embryo research, for example, life was usually considered to begin with "quickening" (feeling the baby move inside the mother) and to end with a dying person's last breath. Now some people argue that life begins with an egg and a sperm in a petri dish and that destroying the resultant embryo is as immoral an act as killing a baby. The common understanding of death has also changed. If a patient stops breathing, doctors can hook up a respirator; if the heart begins to fail, they can transplant a new one. Forty years ago, Barney Clark would never have survived on the strength of his own heart. But the Jarvik-7 gave surgeons power to postpone his death 112 days. Some people believe such a power holds great promise for the future. Others point out that Clark's many operations never improved his health and cost taxpayers millions of dollars. Thus, changing definitions of life and death present society with challenging decisions about who shall live, for how long, and at what cost.

The decisions will be difficult because these situations lack precedents. While many people argue that guidelines can be drawn from traditional sources—religion, philosophy, conscience—others believe these sources do not adequately address what to do about giving a laboratory monkey cancer, creating new life forms from mutant genes, or tipping a few extra embryos down a sink. The situations in which decisions must be made are also highly emotional. Bioethical decisions can mean the difference between having a healthy child or not having one at all, providing a dying stranger with a much-needed organ or keeping a family member alive on life support. While some argue that only doctors and scien-

13

tists should make these decisions, others believe laypeople, especially the families of patients affected by the decisions, should be involved. Thus, *who* should make the decisions becomes as controversial as the decisions themselves.

The chapters in *Biomedical Ethics: Opposing Viewpoints* include: Is Genetic Engineering Ethical? Are Organ Transplants Ethical? Should Limits Be Placed on Reproductive Technology? Should Animals Be Used in Scientific Research? and What Ethical Standards Should Guide the Health Care System? The viewpoints included may not offer answers for cases like that of Barney Clark. It is hoped, however, that they will encourage reflection on ethics, the propriety of technological advances, and the future of human life.

Is Genetic Engineering Ethical?

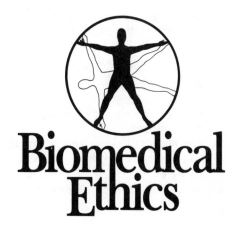

Biomedical
Ethics

"The birth of the gene industry reminds us that . . . innovation is alive and kicking."

Genetic Engineering Will Revolutionize Society

Sharon McAuliffe and Kathleen McAuliffe

Ever since James Watson and Francis Crick discovered the structure of DNA three decades ago, scientists have been experimenting with altering the genetic makeup of living matter to transform plants, animals, and microscopic organisms. In the following viewpoint, Sharon and Kathleen McAuliffe state that this genetic experimentation will prove to be an economic and industrial boon for America. There is no end to the positive things genetic engineering can accomplish—from preventing disease to reconstructing the human brain.

As you read, consider the following questions:

1. What are some of the successes of biotechnology, according to the McAuliffes?
2. Why do the authors believe living beings can be compared to machines?
3. The authors believe genetic engineering may alter our concept of evolution. How? Why do they believe this to be positive?

One chemical holds the secret of life. It contains the instructions for manufacturing everything from a one-celled bacterium to a human being with more than sixty trillion specialized cells. The chemical is called deoxyribonucleic acid, or DNA. It is about to change our world.

In the past few years, dozens of companies have begun to harness the life processes and put them to work in industry. Quietly at first—almost unnoticed in a world dazzled by innovative electronic products—a few pioneering firms set off a technological revolution. It now promises to shake the very foundations of medicine, agriculture, food processing, energy production, and the chemical and pharmaceutical industries.

Success Stories Abound

Biotechnology's success stories already include bacteria engineered to produce human insulin and interferon (the antiviral agent that has hurtled to the forefront of cancer research); a new low-calorie sugar; natural bacterial miners that retrieve copper and uranium; and microbes that pump oil from wells, provide food for livestock, manufacture the main component of antifreeze, and transform industrial pollutants into new sources of energy and starting materials for commercial products.

In the future, biotechnology may bring safe, potent vaccines against everything from malaria and hepatitis to foot-and-mouth, a major disease of livestock; bacteria that break down DDT and other toxic pollutants; and a host of genetically altered plants that will make the supercrops of the Green Revolution seem puny by comparison. Tomorrow's corn and wheat may manufacture their own fertilizers, have vastly improved nutritional value, and flourish without constant pesticide baths.

"The possibilities are so vast that it is impossible to predict the ultimate scope of the impact of recombinant DNA technology," says J. Leslie Glick, the head of Genex, a leading new biology firm. "Suffice it to say that I believe we have observed merely the tip of the iceberg."

What Gregor Mendel, the father of genetics, envisioned as discrete units of heredity more than a century ago have surfaced as a real substance. Genes are synonymous with DNA, a chemical whose structure can now be deciphered, cut, attached to other DNA, and made to work in different organisms. Because DNA is a universal biological language, these recombinant techniques carry across species barriers: human, toad, and bacterial genes can all be joined at will. . . .

Not long ago, experiments with DNA stirred visions of strange, artificial diseases against which humanity would have no natural defense. Such experiments provoked sharp controversy over whether scientists should be allowed to tamper with life itself. Today, those fears have died down—or at least have been pushed to the side. They have been completely overshadowed by reports of the dazzling new products rolling off cell assembly lines and the lucrative gains that await the business community. . . .

Microbes Are Tiny Foot Soldiers

Microbes, or "bugs," as they are affectionately known in the trade, will be the foot soldiers of the biotech revolution. Long before man even suspected the existence of these one-celled creatures, he unwittingly used them in the art of fermentation to make wine, ripen cheese, leaven bread, and pickle various foods. In the twentieth century, fermentation took on a new dimension. Scientists discovered that certain microbes churn out antibacterial agents and began growing them in huge vats. Antibiotics were born, and the age of wonder drugs took off. But of the thousands of microbial strains that exist only a handful have ever been put to work. . . .

Genetic Breakthroughs

The power of recombinant DNA technology lies in the opportunity it offers, for the first time, to produce virtually unlimited quantities of practically any protein. This not only makes possible the production of such things as vaccines and hormones, it also allows biologists to study proteins that up to now were available only in very small quantities.

Ronald W. Ellis, *Science 85*, November 1985.

Once they are located, . . . genetic engineering will often come into play. Scientists will use their tools to improve the bug's natural abilities, to foster the talent of their promising discoveries. Cells often manufacture only small quantities of a desired product, making commercial development impractical. But yields can be stepped up dramatically by inserting multiple copies of a key gene. Yeast has already been engineered to turn out 30 percent more alcohol from corn, an improvement that could soon make fuel-stretching gasohol (a mixture of gasoline and alcohol) competitive in the marketplace. Or several genes found in different microorganisms may be required for a single industrial process. A bug that gobbles up oil slicks was made by fusing the contents of four different bacteria.

Microbes can also be endowed with totally new abilities. Human DNA can be inserted into the genetic machinery of bacterial and yeast cells and made to function. The bugs are tricked into making complex body chemicals never before manufactured by microbes. Until now it has been extremely difficult to extract and purify these substances; only a small percentage have ever been studied or put to clinical use. These inaccessible pharmaceuticals, designed by nature to maintain health and ward off disease, will soon be mass-produced. Gene-spliced drugs are already being tested on human beings and making their way through the Food and Drug Administration's approval process.

Rearranging Cells

Though recombinant DNA is the most powerful tool in the biological revolution, another less sophisticated technique for engineering genes has also attracted commercial interest. Cell fusion, which mixes the entire contents of unmateable cells, was first used to combine two unrelated antibiotic-producing microbes. Their hybrid offspring synthesized a new antibiotic, different from that of either parent strain. Scientists often employ cell fusion when they are unable to identify the genes that code for certain desirable characteristics. It allows them to play a biological crap game. By pushing all the DNA of two cells together, they are gambling on a lucky combination: a hybrid that has inherited the best from both sides of the family.

A variation on this technique enables scientists to turn animal and human cells into immortal antibody factories known as hybridomas. These churn out pure, specific antibodies called monoclonals—weapons the body deploys against foreign invaders and cancerous growths. Antibodies are already used as highly sensitive probes to detect various substances in diagnostic tests. In the future they are likely to play a role in therapeutics, by augmenting the body's natural defense system. While hybridoma technology has grown up in the shadow of recombinant DNA, its impact on medicine is expected to be just as dramatic. . . .

Scientists Can Plan Genetic Changes

The advent of recombinant DNA revolutionizes the way in which genetics can be applied. Scientists no longer have to rely on life's existing properties or try to improve them by inducing random mutations. They can plan the genetic changes, carefully tailoring the organism to meet man's specifications.

In some cases the microbes designed by genetic engineers will provide the only means to obtain a desired product—it is not practical to extract the human body's natural pharmaceuticals, and most are too complex to be synthesized economically. But more often, biotechnology will compete with existing modes of production, providing alternate ways to produce energy, manufacture chemicals, or mine minerals. . . .

The birth of the gene industry reminds us that American innovation is alive and kicking. The nation may lag behind in its older industries, but it hasn't lost its edge with new technologies. Biological processing promises both to save fuel and make renewable energy a feasible alternative to petroleum in the not-too-distant future. By cutting the costs of manufacturing, it could provide a new, noninflationary way to make goods—to reverse the country's alarming productivity statistics. And if properly managed, it offers the opportunity for growth without the pollution problems of today's industry.

Biotechnology makes obsolete the pessimism that pervades our age. Resources are not finite, they are infinitely renewable. Waste is not pollution, it is a source of undreamed-of products and prosperity. It is the realization of the sixties ideal, but with an unexpected twist: technology—the bête noire of the love generation—will bring us back in harmony with the natural order.

The Bases of Man

The growth in our understanding of genetics clearly is revolutionary, with an impact that in the near future may touch each and every one of us. For genes, simply, are the very bases of man.

Jay Stuller, *The American Legion*, January 1984.

Everywhere one looks there is tangible evidence of how physics and chemistry have transformed life in the twentieth century: electricity, plastics, nylon, television, and the computer all remind us of their impact. . . .

Overnight Changes

Now plant, animal, and human genes can be isolated, inserted into plasmids, and grown in bacteria. Overnight the bugs multiply, generating a large mass of cells. This process is known as molecular cloning, since an exact copy of the gene is produced at each division. With a day or two for purification, scientists can easily obtain a milligram of the crucial gene and plenty of its protein product.

The handy plasmid isn't found in higher life forms, so molecular biologists are exploring different types of vectors for transferring new genetic information into plant and animal cells. The aim is to turn breeding into an exact science, where traits are engineered, rather than developed through mating—to transfer genes both across and between species. Basic researchers want to manipulate human and animal cells to reveal the mechanisms that control their growth and development and the malfunctions that bring on disease. Such studies may help to solve both the riddles of cancer (why the DNA of malignant cells somehow goes awry) and aging (cells seem programmed to stop reproducing at a certain point), perhaps enabling us to expand the human life span by decades. . . .

What direction will biotechnology take in the twenty-first century? The answer may be hidden in the theoretical underpinnings of modern biology. As Thomas Kuhn observed, scientific revolutions arise from a conceptual jump in man's thinking—a shift in the basic paradigm or premise that underlies a science. The ideological upheaval that gave birth to molecular biology, and eventually to biotechnology, did not occur overnight. It took several centuries before the mechanistic view of life took hold. How this paradigm emerged and continues to be refined is the best guide to the future.

The central notion—that living organisms are machines—could not have been simpler. Nor is it an accident that it gained popularity as the industrial era arrived in England, when craftsmen became mechanics. Indeed, many of our most fundamental insights about life grew from an understanding of our own mechanical fabrications. The concept of energy, for example, was introduced to explain how water wheels, windmills, and other early machines could be made to do work. Only afterward did scientists come to realize that this concept was equally relevant to the functioning of living organisms. . . .

Over and over again, men have independently converged on nature's solutions to problems. As we began to build machines, the principles we learned gave us insight into the inner workings of life, and we gained a new appreciation for their elegant design. Even our most prized inventions looked crude in comparison to living systems. As our understanding of biology grew, the idea slowly crystallized: why not model our own devices after nature's designs? Why not look first to nature for the answers to technological challenges?

Apprentices to Nature

The discovery of DNA's chemical structure gave this goal validity, and the advent of genetic engineering provided the implements to achieve it. Biomimicry, as the concept has come to be known, is the impetus behind today's revolution in biology. Life is both the raw material and the inspiration for innovation.

At this point, we remain apprentices to nature—and we still have much to learn from her. As novices, we must begin by imitating her craft. Most of our first attempts at bioengineering could not be called original. Existing life forms have been put to work in novel ways, and new life forms have been specially tailored to meet industrial specifications. But most of these modifications represent only minor changes in the basic plan laid down by evolution. Genetically engineered bugs contain less than 1 percent new DNA, and even this genetic material is copied from other living

21

organisms.

Apprentices, however, may themselves become masters in time. Though we are now content to imitate, in the future we will strive to emulate. Our aim is to improve upon nature—to become creators in our own right. Indeed, this trend seems to indicate the general direction in which biotechnology is now headed.

At a . . . conference sponsored by Robert S. First, Inc., leaders of the gene industry explored the exciting possibility of creating enzymes that have no natural counterparts. As more is learned about the active sites of these catalysts and how their amino acid sequences determine the shape and function that characterizes each, scientists may begin designing DNA blueprints from scratch. . . .

Is it really possible to build proteins better than those now in existence? At first glance, this seems highly presumptuous. But to assume otherwise is to deny the course of evolution. Many of the molecules that make up the tissues of living organisms would not have been present in their extinct ancestors. Likewise, the proteins that spring from human ingenuity can be viewed as potential results of evolution in the future. . . .

A New Bionic Animal

Whether tomorrow's computers are fashioned out of proteins or DNA, the outcome is both awesome and unsettling: the brain could be supplanted by a technology born of its own ingenuity. The human species as we know it may be replaced by a new bionic animal that controls its own evolution. A perverse act against man and nature? Perhaps, but from a more cosmic perspective, it might also be viewed as part of the normal (natural?) progression of evolution wherein organisms or their structural components are replaced by the later forms they give rise to in successive stages of adaptation.

Our present definition of technology may be too narrow. The paradigm shift that instigated the biorevolution, in effect, recognized life as a technology. Viewed from this angle, the distinction between man-made machines and living ones blurs. In fact, they may become one and the same. All technologies—whether the opposable thumb, the wheel, or artificial intelligence—are attempts to enhance survival. All are strategies to fight the relentless onslaught of chaos, the entropy that ultimately dooms the universe. That technology should now have a new biological dimension, where man and his inventions interface, could be the inevitable consequence of evolution. Indeed, we may only be seeing evolution at work at a higher level.

We will not attempt a 100-year forecast in the field of biotechnology as a whole. Even our short term predictions are likely to prove conservative. Let it suffice to say that its ultimate potential is mind boggling—and perhaps even mind altering.

"Little or no debate has taken place over the emergence of an entirely new technology that in time could very well pose as serious a threat to the existence of life on this planet as the bomb."

Genetic Engineering May Threaten Humanity

Jeremy Rifkin

With the advent of the technology for bioengineering come vehement arguments against its use. Perhaps the most vocal opponent to bioengineering is Jeremy Rifkin, a political activist, writer, and director of the Foundation on Economic Trends. Rifkin has sponsored numerous successful lawsuits to delay implementation of bioengineering experiments. This viewpoint is taken from his book *Algeny*. Rifkin explains his belief that it is necessary for the survival of humanity as we know it to oppose biotechnological research and development.

As you read, consider the following questions:

1. How does the author suggest that history will be changed by bioengineering?
2. How does Rifkin define eugenics? Why does he believe eugenics is an integral part of biotechnology?
3. Does the author really believe we have a choice between biotechnology and ecology? After reading this viewpoint, do you agree with him?

While the nation has begun to turn its attention to the dangers of nuclear war, little or no debate has taken place over the emergence of an entirely new technology that in time could very well pose as serious a threat to the existence of life on this planet as the bomb itself. With the arrival of bioengineering, humanity approaches a crossroads in its own technological history. It will soon be possible to engineer and produce living systems by the same technological principles we now employ in our industrial processes. The wholesale engineering of life, in accordance with technological prerequisites, design specifications, and quality controls, raises fundamental questions. . . .

Lord Ritchie-Calder, the British science writer, cast the biological revolution in the proper historical perspective when he observed that "just as we have manipulated plastics and metals, we are now manufacturing living materials.". . .

The redesign of existing organisms and the engineering of wholly new ones mark a qualitative break with humanity's entire past relationship to the living world. People's reconception of nature is going to change just as radically as their organization of it. . . .

Our children are beginning to conceptualize the world in a fashion so fundamentally different from anything we can readily identify with that the empathetic association that traditionally passes down through the generations, uniting past with future, seems at times to be irretrievably severed—as if to suggest the termination of one great lifeline in history and the abrupt beginning of another. . . .

Programming Nature

In 1981, the first computerized gene machine made its debut. One need only type out the genetic code for a particular gene on the computer's keyboard and within a matter of a few hours "the machine delivers a quantity of synthetic gene fragments that can be spliced together and put into the DNA of living organisms.". . .

With computer programming of living systems, the very idea of nature being made up of discrete species of living things, each with its own inviolate identity, becomes a thing of the past, a relic of the pre-biotechnical era. Simply by punching in the instructions on a keyboard, it will be possible to cross species walls and program an entire array of novel organisms. Our heirs will live in a world engineered and populated by their own creations. . . .

Living things are no longer perceived as carrots and peas, foxes and hens, but as bundles of information. All living things are drained of their aliveness and turned into abstract messages. Life becomes a code to be deciphered. There is no longer any question of sacredness or inviolability. How could there be when there are no longer any recognizable boundaries to respect? . . .

In the age of biotechnology, separate species with separate names gradually give way to systems of information that can be reprogrammed into an infinite number of biological combinations. It is much easier for the human mind to accept the idea of engineering a system of information than it is for it to accept the idea of engineering a dog. It is easier still, once one has fully internalized the notion that there is really no such thing as a dog in the traditional sense. In the coming age it will be much more accurate to describe a dog as a very specific pattern of information unfolding over a specific period of time. . . .

The New Ethics

A new ethics is being engineered, and its operating assumptions comport nicely with the activity taking place in the biology laboratories.

Eugenics is the inseparable ethical wing of the age of biotechnology. First coined by Charles Darwin's cousin Sir Francis Galton, eugenics is generally categorized in two ways, negative and positive. Negative eugenics involves the systematic elimination of so-called biologically undesirable characteristics. Positive eugenics is concerned with the use of genetic manipulation to "improve" the characteristics of an organism or species. . . .

Abandon DNA Research

"With the splitting of the atom and now with the splitting of the DNA nucleid," says Jeremy Rifkin, "we have reached two technologies that are so inherently powerful, so inherently destructive to our concept of life and the survivability of life, that we best not entertain them. We have a responsibility as a mature species to say 'No,' and to advance our intellectual prowess and our knowledge in areas that are more appropriate to our relationship to the rest of the living ecosystem."

Keenan Peck, *The Progressive*, December 28, 1983.

While the Americans flirted with eugenics for the first thirty years of the twentieth century, their escapades were of minor historical account when compared with the eugenics program orchestrated by the Nazis in the 1930s and '40s. . . .

The new commercial eugenics talks in pragmatic terms of increased economic efficiency, better performance standards, and improvement in the quality of life. The old eugenics was steeped in political ideology and motivated by fear and hate. The new eugenics is grounded in economic considerations and stimulated by utilitarianism and financial gain. . . .

The new commercial eugenics associates the idea of "doing good" with the idea of "increasing efficiency." The difference is that increasing efficiency in the age of biotechnology is achieved by way of engineering living organisms. Therefore, "good" is defined as the engineering of life to improve its performance. In contrast, not to improve the performance of a living organism whenever technically possible is considered tantamount to committing a sin. . . .

No Place To Stop

Proponents of human genetic engineering contend that it would be irresponsible not to use this powerful new technology to eliminate serious "genetic disorders." The problem with this argument, says *The New York Times* in an editorial entitled "Whether to Make Perfect Humans," is that "there is no discernible line to be drawn between making inheritable repairs of genetic defects, and improving the species." The *Times* rightly points out that once scientists are able to repair genetic defects, "it will become much harder to argue against adding genes that confer desired qualities, like better health, looks or brains."

Once we decide to begin the process of human genetic engineering, there is really no logical place to stop. If diabetes, sickle cell anemia, and cancer are to be cured by altering the genetic makeup of an individual, why not proceed to other "disorders": myopia, color blindness, left-handedness? Indeed, what is to preclude a society from deciding that a certain skin color is a disorder?

As knowledge about genes increases, the bioengineers will inevitably gain new insights into the functioning of more complex characteristics, such as those associated with behavior and thoughts. . . . Many sociobiologists contend that virtually all human activity is in some way determined by our genetic makeup, and that if we wish to change this situation, we must change our genes.

Whenever we begin to discuss the idea of genetic defects, there is no way to limit the discussion to one or two or even a dozen so-called disorders, because of a hidden assumption that lies behind the very notion of "defective." Ethicist Daniel Callahan penetrates to the core of the problem when he observes that "behind the human horror at genetic defectiveness lurks . . . an image of the perfect human being. The very language of 'defect,' 'abnormality,' 'disease,' and 'risk,' presupposes such an image, a kind of proto-type of perfection." . . .

The question, then, is whether or not humanity should "begin" the process of engineering future generations of human beings by technological design in the laboratory. What is the price we pay for embarking on a course whose final goal is the "perfection" of the human species? How important is it that we eliminate all the imperfections, all the defects? What price are we willing to pay to extend our lives, to ensure our own health, to do away with all the inconveniences, the irritations, the nuisances, the infirmities, the suffering, that are so much a part of the human experience? Are we so enamored with the idea of physical perpetuation at all costs that we are even willing to subject the human species to rigid architectural design?

With human genetic engineering, we get something and we give up something. In return for securing our own physical well-being we are forced to accept the idea of reducing the human species to a technologically designed product. Genetic engineering poses the most fundamental of questions. Is guaranteeing our health worth trading away our humanity? . . .

As in the past, humanity's incessant need to control the future in order to secure its own well-being is already dictating the ethics of the age of biotechnology. Engineering life to improve humanity's own prospects for survival will be ennobled as the highest expression of ethical behavior. Any resistance to the new technology will be castigated as inhuman, irresponsible, morally reprehensible, and criminally culpable.

The Power To Control

The age of biotechnology will effect a fundamental change in how we govern ourselves. . . .

The power to control the future biological design of living tissue has been signed over to the scientists, the corporations, and the state without ceremony. In return, all that is being asked for are useful products that will enhance human survival and provide for the general well-being.

At first blush, the bargain appears a good one. Biotechnology has much to offer. But, as with other organizing modes throughout history, the final costs have not yet been calculated. Granting power to a specific institution or group of individuals to determine a better-engineered crop or animal or a new human hormone seems such a trifle in comparison with the potential returns. It is only when one considers the lifetime of the agreement that the full import of the politics of the biotechnological age becomes apparent. . . .

Today, the ultimate exercise of power is within grasp: the ability to control the future of all living things by engineering their entire life process in advance, making them a hostage of their own architecturally designed blueprints. Bioengineering represents the power of authorship. Never before in history has such complete power over life been a possibility. The idea of imprisoning the entire life cycle of an organism by simply engineering its organizational blueprint at conception is truly awesome.

In these early stages of the age of biotechnology such power, though formidable, appears so far removed from any potential threat to the human physiology as to be of little concern. We are more than willing to allow the rest of the living kingdom to fall under the shadow of the engineering scalpel, as long as it produces some concrete utilitarian benefit for us. We are even willing to subject parts of our anatomy to bioengineering if it will enhance our physical and mental health. The problem is that biotechnology has a beginning but no end. . . . Thanks to bioengineering, we will finally have been extricated from the great burden of human history, the unremittent need to anticipate and secure our own future. Security will no longer be our concern, because we will no longer control any measure of our own destiny. Our future will be determined at conception. It will be programmed into our biological blueprint. . . .

Era of Danger

We are rapidly moving into a new era of fundamental danger triggered by the rapid growth of genetic engineering. Albeit, there may be opportunity for doing good; the very term suggests the danger. Who shall determine how human good is best served when new life forms are being engineered? Who shall control genetic experimentation and its results which could have untold implications for human survival? . . .

New life forms may have dramatic potential for improving human life, whether by curing diseases, correcting genetic deficiencies or swallowing oil slicks. They may also, however, have unforeseen ramifications, and at times the cure may be worse than the original problem. New chemicals that ultimately prove to be lethal may be tightly controlled or banned, but we may not be able to "recall" a new life form. For unlike DDT or DES—both of which were in wide use before their tragic side effects were discovered—life forms reproduce and grow on their own and thus would be infinitely harder to contain.

Control of such life forms by any individual or group poses a potential threat to all of humanity. History has shown us that there will always be those who believe it appropriate to "correct" our mental and social structures by genetic means, so as to fit their vision of humanity. This becomes more dangerous when the basic tools to do so are finally at hand. Those who would play God will be tempted as never before.

Letter to President Carter from the general secretaries of the National Council of Churches, the Synogogue Council of America, and the United States Catholic Conference, on June 20, 1980.

Two futures beckon us. We can choose to engineer the life of the planet, creating a second nature in our image, or we can choose to participate with the rest of the living kingdom. Two futures, two choices. An engineering approach to the age of biology or an ecological approach. The battle between bioengineering and ecology is a battle of values. Our choice, in the final analysis, depends on what we value most in life. If it is physical security, perpetuation at all costs, that we value most, then technological mastery over the becoming process is an appropriate choice. But the ultimate and final power to simulate life, to imitate nature, to fabricate the becoming process brings with it a price far greater than any humanity has ever had to contend with. By choosing the power of authorship, humanity gives up, once and for all, the most precious gift of all, companionship.

The Choice Is Not Easy

As bioengineering technology winds its way through the many passageways of life, stripping one living thing after another of its identity, replacing the original creations with technologically designed replicas, the world gradually becomes a lonelier place. From a world teeming with life, a world spontaneous, unpredictable, dynamic, rhapsodizing, we descend to a world stocked with living gadgets and devices, a world running smoothly, effortlessly, quietly, without feeling. In the end, it is companionship we give up, the companionship with other life that is at once both indescribable and essential, and without which existence becomes a meaningless exercise. . . .

Our choices, then, are not easy ones. Giving up bioengineering means sacrificing a measure of control over the future. Compromising our drive for total mastery over what lies ahead. Making ourselves more vulnerable so that the rest of existence can become more secure. Choosing to serve and nurture even though we have it in our power to dominate and extract. . . .

Can any of us imagine making such a sacrifice, giving up a measure of control over our own future? Can any of us imagine saying no to all the great benefits that the bioengineering of life will bring to bear? Can any of us, for that matter, entertain even for a moment the prospect of saying no to the age of biotechnology? If we cannot even entertain the question, then we already know the answer. Our future is secured. The cosmos wails.

*"We could be on the threshold not of some
biological utopia but of a catastrophe."*

Genetic Engineering Poses Great Risks

Michael W. Fox

Proponents of genetic engineering promise bigger and more productive farm animals, more effective pesticides, and new disease-
resistant crops. Yet with all the "improvements" come risks.
Michael W. Fox, the director of the Institute for the Study of
Animal Problems and the scientific director of the Humane Society
of the US, argues in the following viewpoint that the risks may
outweigh the advantages. Fox explains that the new pesticides
could cause major ecological imbalances, that bigger and better
animals will be unaffordable and more susceptible to disease, and
that new seeds will not adapt to their biosystems properly. Fox
believes that we must readjust our values or we will be living in
a hazardous environment.

As you read, consider the following questions:

1. Why does the author believe that genetic engineering may
   "disturb the balance and forces of nature"?
2. What risks from genetic engineering does Fox list?
3. Why does Fox believe we may be misusing our power by
   applying biotechnology to animals and crops?

Michael W. Fox, "Genetic Engineering: Cornucopia or Pandora's Box?" *The Futurist*,
February 1986. Reprinted by permission from THE FUTURIST, published by the World
Future Society, 4916 St. Elmo Ave., Bethesda, Maryland 20814.

Genetic engineering is as much a Pandora's box as it is a cornucopia. Without governmental oversight and international coordination to minimize the risks to the environment, we could be on the threshold not of some biological utopia but of a catastrophe.

If we disturb the balance and forces of Nature, disturbances and imbalances will adversely affect the fertility, growth, and fecundity of crops and their primary and secondary consumers—wildlife, farm animals, and human beings. To endeavor to solve food production problems through medical and agricultural bioengineering is to address the symptoms and not the underlying causes.

Genetically engineered microorganisms present new and complex problems for both the environment and for the regulatory agencies that must protect it. The U.S. Environmental Protection Agency (EPA) and other such agencies must now create effective regulations in response to environmental and health concerns.

The EPA has recently decided that bacteria genetically engineered to boost agricultural productivity may be classified as pesticides. Some genetic engineers believe that the new bacterial "pesticides" will quickly die after they have done their work (such as inhibiting frost from forming on potato crops). But these bacteria could cause long-term ecological perturbations because of their influence on other species of bacteria and other living organisms in the environment.

Is This the Right Direction?

Catastrophic possibilities aside, we should ask if we need these new living "pesticides" in the first place. Is this the right direction for agriculture to take?

Many experts insist that it is not, since it is a continuation of capital-intensive farming. What is needed, they argue, is an ecologically sound, regenerative agriculture. The application of genetically engineered bacteria as pesticides is simply a misuse of our power over the gene and over life itself.

For example, genetically engineering certain crops, such as soybeans, to resist some potent herbicide that kills everything else in the fields is a misuse of our power over the gene. While such a package of herbicide and resistant seed could be highly profitable to the manufacturers, drug-dependent farming ultimately is hazardous to all life.

This is not to imply that genetic engineering has no applicability to agriculture. The technique can be used to enhance plants' resistance to drought and disease and to improve crop yields and

31

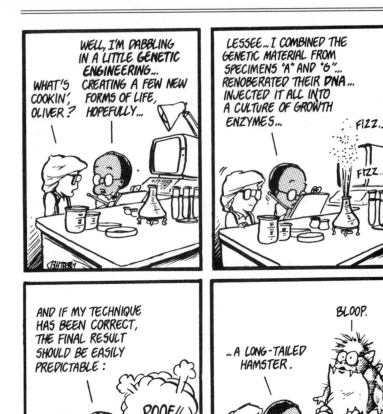

nutrient value.

Genetic engineers have also turned bacteria into biochemical "factories" for the commercial production of vaccines and hormones such as insulin and growth hormone. Such innovations are a significant contribution to the advancement of medicine.

Scientists have recently created giant mice by inserting the growth-regulating genes of rats and humans into them while they are embryos. And this is just the beginning. The U.S. Department of Agriculture is now using this same technique with human genes to create giant pigs and sheep.

Such "super animals" will not feed the world, however. For most of the world's population, meat is a luxury, no matter how "efficiently" the animals are redesigned and managed to turn their feed into protein for human consumption. A de-emphasis on meat production is consonant with an economically and ecologically sound regenerative agriculture.

Proponents of genetic engineering argue that man has, through selective breeding, already modified farm animals to boost productivity. They also argue that these new techniques of gene transfer between species are not fundamentally different from the old method of selective breeding.

This ignores the fact that there are genetic barriers between animal species that prevent interbreeding and the exchange of genes from one species with those from another. This is one of Nature's laws that may be imprudent for us to ignore.

Creating New Problems

Furthermore, selective breeding of farm animals to enhance egg and milk production and growth has contributed to increased susceptibility to infection and new, complex diseases in "factory" farmed animals—so-called production-related or "domestogenic" diseases.

There is also interest in putting genetically engineered bacteria into the digestive systems of farm animals so that they can be used to break down indigestible materials that the animal could not otherwise assimilate and convert into meat, eggs, or milk. But, like spraying new bacterial "pesticides" onto crops, such changes in animals' digestive systems can open Pandora's box further, increasing the likelihood of new disease problems.

Today, the health and well-being of farm animals are sacrificed for overall productivity efficiency and profitability. Tomorrow will be no different, for, as nonrenewable resources (topsoil, water, and fossil fuels) become even scarcer and more costly, the price of animal feedstuffs will increase and farmers will experience even greater economic pressures that will force them to further sacrifice animals' health in order to turn a profit. Those who have "super" animals that grow twice as big twice as fast, or produce more milk or eggs or offspring, will have an economic edge over other farmers who do not have such stock. Another competitive economic treadmill will thus arise.

Regulatory Challenges

The blossoming genetic engineering industry will be regulated by already existing government regulatory agencies. How effective will these agencies be?

The Recombinant DNA Advisory Committee of the National Institutes of Health has established guidelines for research. Some of the committee members believe that the existing guidelines should be abolished, as there have been no accidents or catastrophes involving genetically engineered bacteria since the committee's inception. And . . . the committee ignored its own guidelines by permitting University of California agriculturists to release genetically engineered bacteria into the environment.

No Revolution Without Hazards

"Scientists are not making the distinction between science and technology," argues Sheldon Krimsky, author of *Genetic Alchemy*, a former member of the government's DNA panel, and a professor of urban and environmental policy at Tufts University in Massachusetts. "We have never had a major technological revolution without seeing any hazards associated with it.". . .

Even if there were no cause for great alarm about a possible catastrophe, there is ample reason to worry about the long-term implications of genetic engineering, including questions of environmental impact. Recalling any of the precedents— petrochemical, atomic or plant-breeding industries—is instructive. Chemical engineers in the 1920s and 1930s could not conceive of acid rain even as they worried about explosions; few physicists in the 1940s and 1950s studied the dangers of low-level radiation even as the government considered nuclear accident scenarios; the developers of Green Revolution in the 1960s did not foresee that their high-yield fields would turn out to be more susceptible to blight than conventional ones.

The issue . . . is not so much what can go wrong with genetic engineering but what will happen if everything goes exactly as the engineers plan.

Keenan Peck, *The Progressive*, December 28, 1983.

The EPA will regulate the agricultural applications of biotechnology, as it does the crop-spraying of bacterial pesticides. Manufacturers of bacterial pesticides claim they are safer than regular chemical pesticides. But knowing the public's distrust of pesticides and other agrichemicals, along with its lack of faith in the EPA's ability to effectively monitor and regulate these industries, the EPA will have to collaborate with the biotechnological industries on a massive "public education" public relations campaign, if these new pesticides are to gain acceptance.

Inadequate Regulations

The U.S. Food and Drug Administration (FDA) will regulate new drugs and vaccines developed through biogenetics. But existing FDA regulations and test protocols may be inadequate and inappropriate.

For example, growth hormone manufactured from genetically engineered bacteria passed all routine assays and toxicology tests but was found to have some unanticipated clinical side effects, which were subsequently found to have been caused by unidentified contaminants.

The U.S. Department of Agriculture, which is responsible for the regulation of genetic engineering of plants and animals, faces a difficult task in dealing with the rapidly—and dangerously—shrinking genetic diversity of plants and animals.

Risks of Genetic Engineering

The advent of genetic engineering biotechnology has thrown society into an entirely new dimension wherein we have power over both atoms of matter and the genes of life. How wisely we choose to use this power will depend both on whether we will learn from history and whether we will use newly gained knowledge with both foresight and hindsight.

Some of the risks of genetic engineering include spontaneous mutations and developmental disorders in animals and plants, along with the probability of increased susceptibility to disease. With genetically engineered bacteria, risks include not only the accidental release of harmful organisms, but also problems arising from the deliberately released organisms such as bacterial pesticides. These problems include the survival, multiplication, and dispersal of such bacteria with long-term adverse ecological consequences that cannot be effectively predetermined.

For example, the EPA typically requires small-scale field testing for approval of pesticide products. Chemical pesticides have no independent mobility or reproductive capabilities, and therefore their potential for causing adverse effects outside the treated area is limited.

"Microbial pesticides, however, may replicate and spread beyond the site of application," says an EPA policy statement. "Further, nonindigenous and genetically engineered microbial pesticides may not be subject to natural control or dissipation mechanisms; they may be capable of spreading beyond the site of application with potential adverse effects. Therefore, small-scale field studies with nonindigenous and genetically engineered microbial pesticides would raise many of the same concerns of more extensive use of conventional pesticides."

Rapid development of insect immunity to pesticides—especially if they are highly toxic—and exchange of DNA with naturally occurring bacteria—thus transmitting the traits of genetically engineered microorganisms—are also possible scenarios.

More basic research to allow more accurate prediction of these potential risks is needed if any accurate and valid risk assessments or environmental impact determinations are to be made. Former

EPA chief William Ruckelshaus stated at a recent National Academy of Sciences symposium on biotechnology, "This is the last chance we have to do it right the first time."

Spiral of Instability

Giving seeds insect and disease resistance through genetic engineering will follow a spiral of adaptive instability as insects and diseases gain resistance, mutate, or new pests and diseases appear. Crops cannot be grown in a poisoned and unstable environment. Adaptive stability takes generations of co-evolution (co-adaptation with the soil, climate, other plants, insects, and the rest of the biosystem). Genetic engineering will fail if it continues biologically unstable agricultural practices.

Pathological instability will result from these short-sighted, profit-motivated (or altruistic, though misguided) innovations. For example, genetic engineering to make plants fix nitrogen in the soil themselves, and so not need costly nitrogenous fertilizers, will cause problems if the rate of fixation cannot be regulated by the plant. Nitrate overload could occur, increasing disease and pest susceptibility.

Similar adverse consequences may follow from engineering plants to grow faster or produce more protein. Engineering plants to adapt and grow in hot and cold climates, to which they are not adapted, sounds wonderful. But these plants would be grown in environments where there are insects and diseases with which they have not co-evolved to create a bio-stable relationship and ecology. So more chemicals will be needed to protect them. The residual problems of an improperly applied and inadequately regulated biotechnology industry could become insurmountable— a real-life Pandora's box. . . .

Correct Attitudes Needed

Like putting the cart before the horse, biotechnology will get nowhere if it is not applied within the right conceptual framework. If it is not, there will be crisis after crisis, with the residual problems being caused by one short-sighted step necessitating more genetic tinkering, ad infinitum.

Some may believe that this is the price of progress or high-tech evolution. But consider the myopia of genetic engineering to help crops, livestock, and humans to adapt to a pathogenically disrupted and polluted environment. Which is the first thing that should be corrected? Not the genes, but our attitudes, values, and perceptions.

"The manipulations we're doing in the laboratory are minimal compared with what evolution has done."

Concern Over Genetic Engineering Risks Is Unfounded

David Baltimore: An Interview

David Baltimore earned his Ph.D. in molecular biology at Rockefeller University. A recipient of the Nobel Prize, Baltimore served on the National Institutes of Health Recombinant Advisory Committee which helped guide biotechnology in its early years. Now he is professor of microbiology at MIT, director of the Whitehead Institute for Biomedical Research, and on the board of Collaborative Research, a biotech company. In the following viewpoint, responding to critics, he states that false alarms are creating a bad impression of genetic engineering. He insists that scientists are only mimicking nature and that all experimentation thus far has been thoroughly examined and determined to be safe.

As you read, consider the following questions:

1. Does the author believe that the frost-free bacteria and the livestock viral vaccine are potentially harmful? Why or why not?
2. How does the author equate laboratory experiments with evolution?

"David Baltimore: Setting the Record Straight on Biotechnology" an interview with Alison Bass, *Technology Review*, October 1986. Reprinted and excerpted with permission from TECHNOLOGY REVIEW, M.I.T. Alumni Association, copyright 1986.

Editor's note: In the spring of 1985, a small biotech company, Advanced Genetic Systems, field-tested a genetically altered bacteria without approval from the Environmental Protection Agency. Shortly thereafter, the US Department of Agriculture approved testing for another genetically altered product, a viral vaccine for livestock, without consulting its Recombinant DNA committee. These two incidents generated a public outcry.

TR: As demonstrated by the recent controversies over the field-testing of genetically altered organisms, biotechnology is an area of great concern. Do you think such concerns are valid?

Baltimore: I think genetic engineering in general is something people should be concerned about because molecular biology is extremely potent in what it can do. People ought to be aware of what's going on. However, the two genetically altered products receiving most of the publicity are very poor examples to be concerned about. Both the livestock viral vaccine and the frost-free bacteria are minimal forms of genetic manipulation that will not have a major effect on the environment. That's because the manipulation in both cases involves simply deleting a gene. In the bacteria, scientists deleted a gene that codes for the protein promoting ice formation on plants. Spraying that bacteria on certain crops will protect them against freezing at lower temperatures. In the pseudorabies livestock virus, scientists deleted a gene that makes a protein that apparently contributes to the virus's virulence. When the virus lacks this gene, it can no longer cause disease. It's safe to use as a vaccine strain.

Simple deletions like these occur all the time naturally, and if any one of them produced an organism better adapted to survival than the organism already existing, the mutant organism would have a selective advantage. It would by natural selection become dominant in the environment. So you don't have to worry about a simple deletion of a gene because it has probably already occurred in nature and has been proven not to have a selective advantage. For something to have a major effect on the environment, it has to have a selective advantage over other existing organisms.

TR: Are you saying this "ice-minus" bacteria already exists in nature?

Baltimore: Yes. For all intents and purposes, it does. We don't know that this deletion has occurred in nature in the sense that I can show it to you. We know it in the sense that simple deletions in DNA occur all the time; they occur in human beings.

TR: So why can't we use the mutant bacteria that already exist to protect crops from frost?

Baltimore: If there are a billion bacteria and one of them has this deletion and that deletion is not favored in nature in any way, how do you find it? You can't screen a billion organisms. Also, all mutants look alike. . . . However, it you snip the entire gene out through recombinant DNA methods, there isn't any chance of reversion.

Science Fiction

Some critics fear that certain conjunctions might have potent and unanticipated effects—creating a resistant agent of disease or simply a new creature so hardy and fecund that, like Kurt Vonnegut's *icenine*, it spreads to engulf the earth in a geological millisecond. I am not persuaded by these excursions into science fiction. . . .

We [scientists] have devoted our lives to the study of species in their natural habitats. We have struggled to understand—and we greatly admire—the remarkable construction and operation of organisms, the product of complex evolutionary histories, cascades of astounding improbability stretching back for millions of years. We know these organisms, and we love them—as they are. We would not dissolve this handiwork of four billion years to satisfy the hubris of one species.

Stephen Jay Gould, *Discover*, January 1985.

TR: Does the altered pseudorabies virus exist in nature as well?

Baltimore: Yes. I'm 100 percent sure that a virus with the same thymidine kinase gene deleted in the engineered sequence could be found in nature. And it could be found much more easily than the frost-free bacteria because the genetics of this virus are much better known. I personally don't know why Saul Kit [the researcher who developed the strain] didn't bother trying to find it. I think he was just being fancy and modern in employing recombinant-DNA techniques.

The point is that both these incidents are bad cases: they are cases that ought to be considered routine in a rational world. . . .

The Laboratory and Evolution

TR: Isn't there cause for concern about releasing more complicated genetically altered organisms into the environment—organisms that would not be found naturally and therefore could take over?

Baltimore: We certainly need to examine every case on its merits to decide when concern is reasonable and when it's not. But generally I don't think such organisms will pose a problem for a number of reasons. First, the manipulations we're doing in

39

the laboratory are minimal compared with what evolution has done. Evolution has made you and me out of a bacterium, and we're not doing anything close to that.

TR: But evolution took place over millions, even billions of years and it occurred naturally. Humanity was not in control of evolution the way it is in control of genetic engineering.

Baltimore: That's true. We can work very fast in the laboratory, while natural selection is inevitably a slow process. We can also put together genes from disparate species that don't ordinarily come in contact with one another naturally. So that gives us a new dimension. But whether we're going to do anything fundamentally different and make an organism that is stronger than anything previously seen or more virulent is very doubtful. I think the principles of evolution will hold. It takes very stringent selection to produce something that will do better in a natural environment than what exists before.

TR: If you put a rat growth hormone into a cow, you may not have to worry about that cow adapting to a natural environment. But won't there be some down-the-line effect on the milk supply or something like that?

Baltimore: No. What there will be is a lot more milk from that cow.

Generally Regarded as Safe

TR: But is that healthy for the cow?

Baltimore: No, it's not healthy for that cow. But it's not healthy to be a dairy cow to start off with. And it's certainly not a danger to the environment. For years we have been modifying plants and animals to meet our demands using standard methods of breeding. We have done more to that cow by breeding it over generations than we would by injecting a growth harmone into it.

Let me give you a different example. The difference between a domestic dog and a wild dog is much greater than the differences we're creating in the laboratory—and that difference was created artificially by breeding dogs over generations. How about the nectarine? That's a hybrid between two existing fruits. We've been fooling around with genetics for a long time. When we breed, we fool around with all the genetics available to us through evolution, which is much wider in its variation than the single genes that we manipulate in the laboratory.

TR: Why then aren't people concerned about breeding?

Baltimore: Because it's been going on so long—it's like the GRAS [generally regarded as safe] rule used in regulating pharmaceuticals. Lots of drugs are allowed to be on the market because they were grandfathered in under the GRAS rule. Aspirin, for instance; why hasn't it ever been tested? It was around for a long time before people started worrying about testing.

But the real reason we're not concerned is that none of the new strains has taken over the environment. In fact, all of the new strains are somehow crippled in comparison with the original "wild type."

TR: What is it that makes these artificially created organisms less able to survive naturally?

Baltimore: It's the other way around. What is it that allows something to grow in the wild? It's a conjunction of many traits that allow a plant or animal to get the nutrients it needs, reproduce itself, and live through occasional terrible circumstances such as drought or hurricanes. All of those traits have to be built in, and they're built in by evolution. When you start modifying a plant or animal, you inevitably move away from the optimal solution to something less than optimal.

Genetic Engineering Is Beneficial

The bulk of the [genetic engineering] experiments are not dangerous. They use harmless organisms and produce harmless materials such as human insulin or growth hormone. Of course, if one aims at making a vaccine, one has to use genes from disease-producing organisms. But laboratories will then observe the same precautions that they have always used. . . .

Genetic engineering has now been yielding increasing benefits in medicine, agriculture and industry for six years without causing a day of illness. There is no reason to believe that the novel organisms developed for research or commerce will be more dangerous than the naturally occurring organisms from which they are derived.

Bernard Davis, *U.S. News & World Report,* October 8, 1984.

As a result, the organisms that cause trouble are not the ones that breeder Luther Burbank created and they're not the ones that dog fanciers have bred. The real problem comes with the removal of an organism from its naturally selected environment, away from the pests that control it. That's the really dangerous thing—the starling and gypsy-moth kind of situation. The gypsy moth, which was introduced in the United States in Medford, Mass., from Europe, had no natural predators here, and it went wild because it was extremely well adapted to a natural environment. In some years, gypsy moths eat up a significant fraction of the leaves in forests on the East Coast. . . .

Scientists Regulating Themselves

TR: Because of the controversies over the ice-minus bacteria and the viral vaccine, some people have compared the nascent biotech industry to the nuclear power industry two decades ago.

Baltimore: Boy is that a mistake. First of all, the biotech industry has taken into account public concerns in a meaningful way—right from the beginning. That was certainly not true in the nuclear power industry or in any other industry. In this case a group of people raised questions about whether everything was safe at the first signs of a powerful new technique, and asked that a decision be made by a governmental body about what was appropriate and how we should go forward. It was technology assessment at the very inception of the technology—and that is highly unusual in this country.

TR: Are you referring to the moratorium on recombinant-DNA experimentation that the scientists themselves called for in the mid-1970s?

Baltimore: Yes. A number of us within the scientific community met here at M.I.T. and drafted what is known as the Berg letter [Nobel laureate Paul Berg chaired the group]. That letter asked that scientists not carry out certain kinds of experiments until some experts could really look at them and see whether they were safe. That generated a moratorium and at the conference at Asilomar [in California], we drafted rough guidelines and a mechanism for making sure recombinant-DNA experiments were carried out in a safe and appropriate manner. From that conference, NIH [National Institutes of Health] guidelines evolved and the Recombinant Advisory Committee (RAC) was set up to review and approve research experiments involving recombinant DNA. RAC was also intended to modify the guidelines as knowledge about the field grew.

Concerned About Safety

TR: So how would you say RAC was different from, say, the Nuclear Regulatory Commission?

Baltimore: First of all, it was a voluntary review process. Molecular biologists in academia and industry voluntarily submitted themselves to the RAC jurisdiction from the beginning. That meant that the whole biotechnology industry developed within the context of concern about safety. To my knowledge, everyone in the industry was aware of that concern and was responding to it. . . .

TR: What specifically would have been inhibited by rigid regulation in the early 1980s?

Baltimore: A perfect example was the cloning, sequencing, and characterization of animal viruses—that is, identifying the viral genes and finding out what they do and how they're organized. This research was held up for a number of years because its original classification by RAC required extremely high containment facilities. Very few labs had such facilities. As a result, no work was done on viruses until we discovered that such research was safe to do without extreme precautions and modified the guideline. If the original classification had been written into law, viral research would have been stalled for a much longer time. Once you make a law, it's very hard to change it.

TR: Can you give me a specific example of something constructive that came out of the viral research allowed by RAC?

Baltimore: The understanding of the AIDS virus. Scientists were able to identify the causative agent of AIDS rapidly because we knew so much about this kind of virus, largely as a result of recombinant-DNA work. . . .

Intense Discussion

TR: People are still having second thoughts. Aside from the issue of environmental release, some critics are saying that the scientific community is rushing pell mell into human gene therapy without considering the enormous ramifications of such treatment. Do you agree?

Baltimore: The scientific community has been intensively discussing the ramifications of human gene therapy for five years at a minimum, and I can remember discussions going back to the 1960s. The community has thought about this issue for years. I myself spend an inordinate amount of time talking with people about it. The public debate is in the newspapers every week in one form or another. In 1982, a presidential commission studied the issue in depth. The group wrote a report that drew a strong line between "somatic-cell" therapy, which involves implanting a normal gene into the body cells of a patient with a serious disorder, and "germline" therapy, which involves inserting a new gene into the reproductive cells that are passed onto future generations. No one is presently considering doing germline therapy. The presidential commission said that we should go ahead with somatic therapy as long as we know the treatment is effective and the patient has a serious disorder.

Since then, RAC has published guidelines on how the first somatic-gene therapy should be handled. There are still technical difficulties to work out, and I don't think we're going to see attempts at human gene therapy for a year or more. It seems to me that we have developed this new capability in a very deliberate manner. When media people or government officials think something is happening very fast, I think it is often because they are not aware of the extent of the preceding debate.

43

"The safety record for . . . genetic engineering indicates that little or no additional regulation is necessary."

Government and Science Can Adequately Regulate Biotechnology

Ralph W.F. Hardy and David J. Glass

Ralph W.F. Hardy, a biochemist, is president of BioTechnica International and a visiting professor at Cornell University. David J. Glass received his Ph.D. in biochemical sciences from Princeton University. He is director of patents and regulatory affairs at BioTechnica International. In the following viewpoint, Hardy and Glass write that genetic engineering techniques, though controversial, are essentially safe and will provide benefits for medicine, agriculture, and other industries. They argue that excessive regulation will stifle business and research causing the US to lose the lead it has over its international competitors. They believe that current scientific and government regulations adequately handle the biotech industry.

As you read, consider the following questions:

1. Why do the authors believe that genetic engineering technologies are safe?
2. How do safety issues affect genetic engineering regulations, according to the authors?

Ralph W.F. Hardy and David J. Glass, "Our Investment: What Is At Stake?" *Issues in Science and Technology*, Spring 1985. Copyright by National Academy of Sciences, 2101 Constitution Avenue, Washington, DC 20418. Reprinted by permission.

The United States is spending $1.5 billion a year, from both public and private sources, to develop the new technologies of genetic engineering. By all accounts the benefits of genetic engineering are expected to be substantial. They will include new technology and products for a variety of major industries, including health care, agriculture, energy, and pollution control. In the health care field, genetic engineering may provide new approaches for treating cancer and cardiovascular disease, major killers in the industrialized world. Genetic engineering will also increase food production, and may thereby aid in averting famines in developing nations. Current sales of genetic engineering products are modest but are expected to climb to more than $100 billion in the year 2025. States, cities, and the federal government are aggressively trying to provide the climate that will attract and foster strong genetic engineering industries.

The United States is now the world leader in genetic engineering, but international competition is increasing. A major factor in determining the continued strength of the U.S. position will be regulation of the new genetic engineering industries. Questions of safety have arisen recently, particularly concerning the release of genetic engineering products into the environment. However, there is no reason to suspect that these new applications of genetic engineering will pose significant risks. Moreover, unrealistic regulation could impede the ability of U.S. industries to maintain their current lead in genetic engineering. If this opportunity is not to be lost, regulations must be appropriate, and should be based on considerations of the record of negligible risk from genetic engineering to date, as well as on perceived risks and benefits. . . .

Regulatory Concerns

Several factors will be important to the success of the cellular and molecular genetic engineering industry. Genetic engineering technologies have been controversial from the start, and the industry will have to make an effort to achieve public acceptance of its goals. Ethical, religious, and moral concerns still trouble a segment of the population, as does the issue of safety. In addition, in proposing sweeping changes in world agriculture, the industry must consider a number of questions. For example, will genetic engineering harm the genetic diversity of the world's crops? What will be the effect of improved food, nutrition, and health care on world population and the quality of life?

Other factors of a more technical nature are important to the industry's success as well. Adequate financing is essential if companies are to develop products and see them through the

regulatory, manufacturing, and marketing processes. This requirement has led to a search for creative financing approaches.
Although R&D tax credits assist profitable established companies
in funding genetic engineering activities, such credits are of no
use to start-up companies during their critical early years. How
can government support the activities of the start-up companies,
which may be the key to U.S. industrial strength in genetic
engineering? In addition, industry must maintain a good relationship with the academic community, both because continuing basic
research is critical to the industry and because universities are
responsible for training future scientists and engineers.

Use Existing Laws

Federal regulations of field testing and commercialization of the
products of biotechnology should be effective, scientifically based
and implemented under existing laws. . . .

Safety and environmental tests have for years been an integral part
of our development program of the altered microbe. We've studied
the microbes to understand their physiology.

We've looked for effects on other organisms on land and in water
and found none. We've devised ways to monitor the microbe in
the soil. And we've developed ways to destroy it, if necessary. . . .

As an industry, we already see vigorous competition emanating from
Europe and Japan. West Germany, Japan and the United Kingdom
each have federally supported biotechnology institutes.

Field testing of agriculture products *will* be permitted in the United
States.

It is only a matter of time. When the American farmer is ready to
buy high-performance crop seeds and microbial pesticides, will he
have to turn to suppliers in Japan or Europe? Why shouldn't we,
the American industries that serve agriculture and the American
farmer and the American consumer, become the beneficiaries of
genetic engineering?

Will D. Carpenter, *Los Angeles Times*, April 27, 1986.

Patent protection is also of prime importance. Will genetically
engineered products be protectable under the U.S. and foreign
patent systems? Will additional protection become available
through legislative reform—for example, in patent-term restora-
tion and process-patent infringement? Another issue is whether
current government policy will foster the growth of the industry,
enabling the United States to maintain its lead. Several policies
of the federal government come into play here, such as those involving the export of unapproved new drugs and the broader issue

of more realistic government regulation.

The issue of government regulation to protect human health and the environment is perhaps of the most immediate concern to industry. If excessive, regulation can cause significant delays in product development, at a cost that can be catastrophic for small companies. Yet the regulation of genetic engineering is once again the subject of national debate, with many of its proponents stating an intent to "do it right this time" by agreeing on adequate regulatory oversight in the industry's early years.

No Evidence of Hazard

It is worth noting that the proposed regulation of the biotechnology industry is unique. If regulations are imposed, this would be one of the few cases in which an industry has been made subject to significant health and safety controls before any hazards have been proved or any industrial accidents have occurred. Indeed, after nearly 10 years of close scrutiny, risk-assessment studies, and worldwide experience with molecular and cellular genetic manipulations, there is no evidence of any significant hazards associated with this technology—the risks remain only speculative. In fact, with the accumulation of knowledge, many of the fears voiced in the early days of molecular genetics have been shown to be unfounded.

Furthermore, there is no reason to believe that cellular and molecular genetic engineering should present any greater hazard than that posed by the whole organism genetic engineering that has been practiced for centuries. If anything, in light of the directed nature of the changes introduced into organisms through molecular genetic engineering, the possible adverse effects of modified organisms can be more reliably predicted than those associated with organisms mutated by traditional breeding.

... the new technologies of cellular and molecular genetic engineering differ from whole organism engineering mainly in the methods used to produce the desired genetic variation, as well as in applications and knowledge about genetic changes. It would seem logical that the method of producing the genetic variation would be less important that the end product in terms of possible deleterious effects on human health or the environment. On that basis, the products of whole organism, cellular, and molecular engineering should be similarly regulated.

For a number of reasons, however, products of molecular genetic engineering have drawn special attention that may lead to an increased regulatory interest in the coming years. This will especially involve those microorganisms and plants modified by molecular techniques and designed for use in the environment, including modified crop plants and microbes designed to clean up oil spills, to improve crop nutrient supply, to protect crops against frost damage, and to act as pesticides. Concern has been raised that in the course of small-scale field tests, the modified organisms might multiply unchecked and have adverse environmental effects.

Public Concern

Increasingly, the public perceives that the risks posed by small-scale field tests are real and that neither government nor industry is equipped to assess them. What is often ignored, however, is that in most cases the new organisms are similar either to genetically engineered organisms already in commercial use or to naturally occurring organisms indigenous to habitats where they would be used. In these cases, experience with the wild-type or mutated organisms provides information with which to access the potential risks of the new organisms. Indeed, the fact that similar organisms exist or have been previously introduced into the environment suggests that no adverse effects would occur from the introduction of a novel strain.

No Societal Evaluation Needed

The major concerns about genetic engineering have been debated, tracked and extensively analyzed beginning 10 years ago, when science began to use these techniques. The committee at the National Institutes of Health regulating recombinant DNA research established strict rules in the mid-1970s for such work but made provisions for relaxing them if possible. What we have learned from all this experience and analysis is that the fears were unfounded. No environmental or health problems from this research have occurred, and the NIH rules have been opened up. . . .

National Institutes of Health scientist Maxine Singer wrote, "Societal evaluation, . . . which in our country means legislative or judicial review, is bound to be unwise, even tragic, unless it is based on facts rather than fantasies." The government-wide rules signed by Mr. Reagan are expected to make a key recognition of reality, by greatly reducing the current regulatory burden on gene-deleted products such as the pseudorabies vaccine and the frost-preventing bacteria.

The Wall Street Journal, May 23, 1986.

In addition, the techniques of molecular genetics also provide a method to monitor the distribution of the engineered genes in the environment. Pieces of DNA complementary to introduced genes or to a signature sequence of DNA coupled to the introduced genes can now be used in the laboratory to probe for organisms carrying added DNA. In time it will be possible to use this DNA probe technology to facilitate monitoring in the field.

In light of these public concerns, industry has recognized that some regulation of the environmental applications of genetic engineering is necessary. Although no new laws or regulations are needed, the recent debate has illuminated areas in which existing regulatory authority may be better exercised to apply to the products of the new genetic methodologies. Discussion has also centered on the need for better risk-assessment tools.

Industry desires a stable, realistic regulatory regime. Such a regime would allow companies developing products for release into the environment to incorporate the time and cost required to meet regulatory requirements into their strategic planning. Unrealistic regulations that impede progress will not be well received by industry. Moreover, in the face of increasing international competition, the United States risks losing its competitive edge if the biotechnology industry is regulated too stringently. The start-up companies face an additional burden. This valuable U.S. resource could be severely damaged or lost if unrealistic regulations are established or regulatory agencies move slowly. Unlike many established companies, start-up companies do not have the financial reserves to withstand major delays before marketing a product.

Regulatory Recommendations

The following general recommendations could provide a basis for constructing an appropriate regulatory regime:

- *Use existing laws.* Products of cellular and molecular genetic engineering could be covered by existing laws. This approach would avoid the confusion of writing new laws for unknown risks.
- *No additional regulatory requirements are necessary for cellular and molecular genetic engineering.* There are no special risks inherent in the cellular and molecular genetic engineering technologies that compel additional requirements in the regulatory process. These processes should be seen as alternative manufacturing methods, and risk analysis should focus on the end products rather than on the processes.
- *Government agencies should have clear jurisdiction over discrete product areas.* Duplication of regulatory authority will lead to unnecessary disputes and delays.
- *Proper scientific review.* Risk-assessment studies must be based on case-by-case review by qualified scientists. Agencies should rely on outside consultants in the short term if this expertise is not available in-house, but they should quickly establish in-house capabilities.
- *Use the available risk record from whole organism engineering.* There has been considerable experience with the products of whole organism engineering in commerce and in the environ-

ment. This record should be considered in conducting risk-benefit analyses of the products of cellular and molecular genetic engineering.

- *Research needed.* Government agencies should conduct or sponsor further research to develop the information and the risk-assessment tools that are perceived to be needed.
- *Society should directly bear the costs.* Regulation proposed for genetic engineering is unique in that there are no proven hazards or industrial accidents related to the technology. Thus, there is every reason why society—not industry—should shoulder the burden of this regulation.

In sum, the safety record for whole organism genetic engineering indicates that little or no additional regulation is necessary for cellular and molecular engineering. In fact, the directed approach made possible by molecular genetic engineering is further evidence of its safety. Only in these new technologies is it possible to know and control the exact nature of the genetic change, unlike the more random processes used for years in breeding and selection. Moreover, it is becoming possible to fashion probes to monitor the fate of new genetic constructions, and biocides can be developed to recall novel organisms from the environment. Some regulation, however, appears to be inevitable. If these regulations are developed from a realistic assessment of risks and benefits, then industry should be able to maintain its competitive edge in this promising new field. If they are overly stringent, both a major dollar and talent investment and an economic opportunity will be lost.

"Whatever regulatory method is chosen, it must make provisions for public involvement."

Government Biotechnology Controls Are Not Sufficient

Gina Maranto

As more and more companies move into the biotechnology business, they encounter mistrust from public interest groups and politicians. Many people argue that scientists, biotech executives, and government regulatory committees have tended to ignore the fears of the outside community and push for their own special interests. In the following viewpoint, Gina Maranto, a writer for *Discover*, a popular science magazine, concludes that the biotech industry must earn the trust and support of the public if it is to continue to develop.

As you read, consider the following questions:

1. According to the author, what most worries opponents of the biotechnology industry?
2. What suggestions does Maranto offer for public involvement in regulating biotechnology?
3. What are some reasons, according to Maranto, for lack of public involvement in the biotech industry?

Gina Maranto, "Genetic Engineering: Hype, Hubris, and Haste," *Discover,* June 1986. © *Discover* Magazine. Reprinted by permission.

Suddenly, gene technology, a subject that had lately been relegated to the business section of your newspaper, was back on the front page. First, on Feb. 26, [1986], it was reported that Advanced Genetic Sciences Inc. (AGS) had illegally tested a genetically altered bacterium by injecting it into fruit and nut trees on the roof of its headquarters in Oakland, Calif., nine months before the Environmental Protection Agency (EPA) granted the company a permit to test the microbe outside the laboratory. Advanced Genetic's defense was feeble: the microbes hadn't really been released into the environment because they were contained within the trees. Then, on April 3, came more shocking news: without informing anyone, the U.S. Department of Agriculture (USDA) had on Jan. 16 granted the Omaha-based Biologics Corp., a subsidiary of the Tech-America Group Inc., a license to market a genetically engineered vaccine for pseudo-rabies, a deadly disease that afflicts pigs, cattle, and sheep. In contravention of federal policy, the USDA had also issued a permit for testing the vaccine outside the laboratory. Biologics scientists used the new vaccine on 1,000 three-day-old pigs in four Midwestern states. There's some question whether the company fully explained the implications of the vaccine to the state agriculture departments involved until six months subsequent to the tests. One week after the Biologics story broke, the USDA suspended the license—to get its paperwork in order, it said. On April 22 it was re-issued, whereupon Jeremy Rifkin filed suit. At a congressional hearing on the matter a week later, there was finger pointing all around, after a committee that reviews genetic engineering research at Texas A & M faulted the researchers involved for sidestepping federal rules by performing newly disclosed outdoor tests in 1984. . . .

Government Approach Light-Handed

The AGS and USDA episodes occurred as several biotech products were about to move out of the lab and into the marketplace, and they lent weight to charges made over the past few years by a widening circle of critics—including historians and philosophers of science, public interest groups, politicians, and scientists—that the federal government's approach to regulating genetic engineering has been too light-handed. While agreeing that biotechnology is likely to benefit society in the long run, these critics question the wisdom of rushing to release live altered microbes before fully considering the environmental consequences.

What worries them most is the prospect that biotechnology's products, like those of past technologies, may wreak changes that

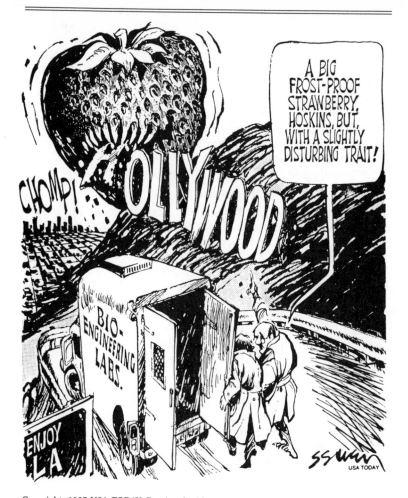

cannot be foreseen—and perhaps, at first, not even measured. There's no science of predictive ecology, so any assessment of the hazards of gene-spliced organisms is largely speculative. The risk of an Andromeda strain arising is probably minimal, but there's reason for exercising caution. As the eminent biochemist Erwin Chargaff, a professor emeritus at Columbia, said, "You cannot recall a new form of life." Since scores of genetically engineered products are expected to be ready for marketing or field-testing in the next five years, many critics think safeguards must be instituted now, before, as one skeptic says, "a mini Three Mile Island happens."

Critics charge, in addition, that those guiding the new industry are ignoring social and political issues. The picture they paint is of an industry beset by financial difficulties and eager to avoid further delays that might worsen its image among investors, and of an administration dedicated to easing the industry's way and giving the public less of a role in making biotechnological decisions. Groups like the Boston-based Committee for Responsible Genetics, whose board of advisers includes more than a dozen leading biologists, have contended for some time that questions concerning the impact of biotechnology on universities and society at large haven't been adequately addressed by either the companies engaged in gene splicing or the government.

Ice-Minus Case

In the minds of some biotech watchers, the contention that things are moving too rapidly was borne out in the AGS case. In November, against the advice of soil agronomist Martin Alexander of Cornell, one of its most respected advisers, the EPA granted AGS a permit to spray a strawberry patch in Monterey County with a genetically altered strain of *Pseudomonas* bacterium, called ice-minus, that greenhouse tests have shown will forestall frost formation on the plants. . . . Local residents, alarmed by the prospect of the AGS test, petitioned the Monterey County board of supervisors, which voted twice to block the spraying of the strawberry patch. At a packed public hearing in January, county residents angrily accused AGS, state officials, and the EPA of negligence: no one from the company or the government agencies had informed them of the planned release; instead they learned about it from national television and radio. . . .

After a hasty investigation, the EPA revoked the ice-minus permit and levied the maximum penalty, $20,000, for the wrongdoing—which the company admitted to, although it claimed it had not falsified documents, as charged. The agency left open the possibility that AGS could still carry out the test after conducting further safety studies and winning a second permit.

An Impatient Industry

Just days after the Advanced Genetic permit was granted, a spokeswoman for the Committee for Responsible Genetics fired off an angry letter to Steven Schatzow, director of the pesticides section of the EPA: "The recent approval sends a signal that the agency has abandoned its initial 'proceed with caution' approach in deference to the wishes of an impatient biotechnology industry."

Senator Albert Gore Jr. (D-Tenn.), who's of the opinion that biotechnology shouldn't be "unduly impeded," also registered displeasure. "I think this experiment is almost devoid of significant risk to the environment," he said. "But the procedure used for approving it is totally inadequate, and future proposed experiments will require the sort of information [on how the microbe might spread] that was waived as a requirement this time." Gore later said, "If the administration cannot come up with a workable solution, the Congress may do it for them.". . .

Cultural Schizophrenia

Grass roots fear of gene splicing is running high. After the EPA approved ice-minus, picketers carrying NO GENETIC MANIPULATION placards marched in front of AGS headquarters, and opponents in Monterey began drafting a county law covering releases of genetically altered microbes. Missouri environmental groups have voiced concerns about a proposed outdoor test in that state by the Monsanto Corporation of an engineered soil bacterium carrying a gene for a protein toxic to insects. And in April, Wisconsin dairy farmers, alarmed by predictions that 20 to 30 percent of dairy owners will be forced out of business within three years after the licensing of a hormone that boosts milk production in cows, called on the Food and Drug Administration (FDA) to take a closer look at the drug.

No Public Involvement

The whole field of biotechnology is shrouded in mystery. There is virtually no public involvement in biotech development and, as yet, no set policies to guide it. It appears that most biotech research is being conducted by private companies. Society can influence private research through government regulatory agencies or the courts. Both of these methods are after-the-fact controls at best.

Technology is a strong tool for social planning; the public should be able to discuss and then influence the direction of technological development. The public needs to take back some control and responsibility for developing the kind of future it wants. . . .

Technology ought to adapt to people instead of the other way around.

Richard Ness and Ruth Tonachel, *Minneapolis Star and Tribune*, July 6, 1986.

Genetic engineering has engendered a certain amount of cultural schizophrenia from the outset. When it was first brought to the public's attention in the early 1970s, the new biology was billed as having the power to solve just about any global problem, including pollution, desertification, hunger, and disease. In some respects that view persists. A presidential committee on biotechnology spoke for scientists and businessmen alike when in 1984 it said, "The tremendous potential of biotechnology to contribute to the nation's economy in the near term, and to fulfill society's needs and alleviate its problems in the longer term, makes it imperative that progress in it be encouraged."

But if genetic engineering was the stuff of Utopian Studies 101, it was also the stuff of Faust and Frankenstein. James Watson, who shared a Nobel Prize for the discovery of the structure of DNA, has recounted how scientists in the early '70s started to fear what they had found: "We began to ask whether in the process of possibly discovering the power of 'unlimited good,' we might simultaneously be setting the stage for discovering the power of 'unlimited bad.'". . .

Public Fears

Says one critic, "People haven't bought the notion that this technology is nothing but good, that we don't have to worry about it and should plough ahead."

Lack of public confidence in genetic engineering could mean that biotech firms will be tied up in litigation for years. What's needed to avert such a situation, say many observers, is a concerted effort by industry and government to evaluate risks to health and the environment, and to address other public concerns. "If the biotechnology industry is to flourish," Senator Gore says, "it must have the support of the people of this country. The industry won't be able to survive if the public fears it.". . .

Engineered Organisms

Most ecologists just want to see the industry properly monitored. In a letter to *Science* . . . , five prominent environmental researchers wrote: "We neither doubt the great potential for benefits resulting from the ability to move genes between unrelated species, nor do we believe that most plans for such projects would have severely harmful ecological impacts. We would argue, however, that even traditional breeding has not been ecologically trouble-free, that engineered organisms are analogous to exotic [imported or transplanted] ones to some extent, and that the particular kinds of engineering that are now contemplated are quite likely, if inadequately regulated, to lead to some instances of ecological harm."

Molecular biologists have insisted that altered organisms can hardly cause trouble when they're released, because in most cases researchers merely remove, replace, or add one gene in modifying a microbe or plant. Similar mutations continually arise in bacterial populations in the wild without causing problems, they claim.

This argument was used by David Kingsbury, the National Science Foundation's assistant director for biological, behavioral, and social sciences, to explain why the animal and plant health inspection service had treated Biologics' pseudo-rabies vaccine like any other vaccine. He said that since the new vaccine was made simply by deleting one gene from an already approved vaccine, it "didn't fall within the regulatory guidelines.". . .

At the National Science Foundation building on Washington's G Street, . . . Robert Rabin, assistant director for life sciences in the President's Office of Science and Technology Policy, talked with Kingsbury about why Congress should stay out of the biotechnology business.

Kingsbury: You certainly can retard this industry by legislating regulations. The Delaney Clause [which says that drugs showing any evidence of being carcinogenic must be treated as carcinogenic] is an example of how one can run amuck. You're guilty until proved innocent.

Social Impacts

The White House plan, which seeks to minimize interference in the biotech industry, has been criticized by some public interest groups on the grounds that it overlooks risks posed by this new technology to the public health and environment. . . .

According to Sheldon Krimsky, professor of Environmental Policy at Tufts University and a former member of RAC, "the most important problems are not technical problems. The decision to develop a technology in a certain direction is a social concern with important social impacts. Decisions will be made by default without a broad examination that transcends the narrow focus of the [federal] agencies. The structure right now is designed to speed up industrialization of biotechnology."

Samantha Sparks, *Multinational Monitor*, February 28, 1986.

Rabin: If we apply the same thing to this game, we're going to make it infinitely more difficult not only for industry but also for researchers.

Kingsbury: If we approach biotechnology as if it's dangerous until we prove that it's not, we'll never prove it's not, and we'll never go anywhere.

In the modern era, regulation may have slowed the march of science and technology, but it hasn't prevented them from going anywhere. For example, the petrochemical industry has been heavily regulated and has nonetheless flourished: it now produces 8,000 chemicals.

While neither Rabin nor Kingsbury claims that the biotech industry is vital to the U.S. economy, they agree that it's important enough that clearly defined—and none too stringent—regulations should quickly be put in place. Other federal officials have also argued that the government has a duty to help speed genetic engineering along by determining just what's expected in the way of pre-market tests and environmental impact analyses—if not by extending economic incentives. They maintain that the Japanese, the West Germans, the British, and the French have given high priority to biotech, and any bureaucratic tie-ups here could jeopardize the world leadership of U.S. firms. Since biotechnology promises enormous economic and social benefits and poses few risks, they say, there's even more reason not to delay.

Many experts dispute such reasoning; they contend that biotechnology's putative benefits are pie in the sky and shouldn't be used to justify an easing of regulations. Some even say it would be no great loss to the world if many of the products now in the pipeline never reached the market. . . .

How To Regulate

How, or whether, to regulate the industry remains a major issue. Sheldon Krimsky [an associate professor of urban and environmental policy at Tufts] divides the opinion into four camps. There's the conservative, free enterprise, don't-regulate-until-you-see-the-whites-of-their-eyes camp—a small minority. "Forget the hazards," they say. "Let's push on." There's the camp that says, "Let's have reasonable regulations and proceed." Then there are the critics that say, "Let's negotiate our demands. Where the process will end, we can't tell. Society will make the ultimate decision." Last, there's the camp that says, "Let's not proceed at all," and will use any legal technique to obstruct the industry's activities. . . .

The Reagan administration falls between the first camp and the second. While it's opposed to the drafting of new laws to regulate biotechnology, of late it has moved toward putting biotech under existing federal statutes. . . .

No Public Input

In October [1985] the Biotechnology Science Coordinating Committee (BSCC) was chartered under the President's Office of Science and Technology Policy to facilitate regulation of the industry. Its stated purpose is to foster consistency and cooperation among the various agencies involved. . . .

Part of the role of the BSCC seems to be to allay public fears, which, depending on your view, can be salutary or insidious. Rabin and Kingsbury suggest that the BSCC, of which Kingsbury is chairman, may diminish the power of the NIH's recombinant DNA committee. Although administration officials say the recombinant DNA panel has no statutory authority and simply couldn't handle the fast-paced biotech industry, others say the real motive for sidestepping it was to move the decision making on genetic engineering further out of the public arena. Says Krimsky, who sat on the recombinant DNA committee from 1979 to 1981, "The BSCC has no public members, can proceed with almost no outside input, and offers little public access. It can be seen as nothing more than a system to ease the regulatory process for an industry that's finding it increasingly difficult to gain the confidence of the investment community."

Biotech executives now seem resigned to what's happening at the federal level. Two years ago there were those who thought companies could avoid regulation, and those who felt they could live with regulation—if they only knew what form it would take. Now the latter view prevails, and insiders realize they were mistaken to assume that biotechnology would be exempt from supervision. Says [Thomas] Dyott [AGS president], "When biotechnology was first coming onto the horizon, a lot of people contrasted it with the—in their minds—sinister chemical industry. Since biotechnology was about life processes, presumably its products would be biodegradable. So they thought that biotechnology would be virtually free of regulation. But it was naive to expect that biotechnology is so clean that no one would have questions about it, and that it wouldn't require regulations.". . .

Growing Resistance

The Federal regulators' apparent uncertainty about every announced field test or field-test plan has resulted in widespread suspicion among the public, and as a result several communities have established their own regulations. Monterey County, California, banned tests on ice-minus for months. These actions resemble the growing local resistance to other potentially dangerous technologies, such as nuclear waste disposal.

Charles Pillar, *The Nation*, October 25, 1986.

Members of the camp that wants to negotiate on biotech say that whatever regulatory method is chosen, it must make provisions for public involvement. The Committee for Responsible Genetics advocates public representation at all levels of the review process, which presumably means in the federal agencies as well as on the BSCC—or any similar committee that might be created. Other experts recommend a plural system, with national and local regulatory bodies all having public members. "It would be messy," says Everett Mendelsohn, [a Harvard historian of science], "but in a democratic society a lot of things are messy. It would give you a way to slow things down so that people would have a chance to ask what values they were trading off—scientific for democratic, democratic for scientific—at each point along the way.". . .

Public Scrutiny

The thought of intense public scrutiny strikes many scientists as distasteful. Watson once voiced dismay that "public members [of review boards] may take regulation seriously, unlike the molecular biologists." Some critics say this attitude isn't surprising, considering what researchers have at stake. But indications are that if the public were to get involved on a large scale, the progress of research in university or commercial labs wouldn't necessarily be slowed. In 1982 Diana Dutton, a senior research associate at Stanford, surveyed the records of 20 biosafety committees in California that monitored biotechnology experiments at academic and industrial labs. She found that during the year studied, 1979, committees with public members reviewed almost twice as many research proposals as those with none.

The position that non-scientists couldn't master enough of the complexities of DNA and monoclonal antibodies and bioprocessing to do a competent job of assessing the risks—a claim sometimes made by the experts—isn't borne out by events. When people feel threatened, they manage to learn a great deal. "My point of departure is medicine," says Halstead Holman [an M.D. who teaches internal medicine at Stanford]. "I have the privilege of seeing real people of all backgrounds addressing themselves to the intrusion of technology into their lives and making decisions about whether they will allow a test, allow a treatment, and so on. There's no question in my mind that average citizens deal with these problems very well. . . .

Mendelsohn has a more trenchant reply to experts who say the issues are too tough for the rest of us to comprehend. "If any scientific or technical project is so complicated that the lay public can't understand it when it's explained," he says, "then it shouldn't be done. If it is done, then we've ceded our responsibility for critical decision making to a select élite. No democratic society can tolerate that."

Society Should Decide

Commercialism represents a far more powerful influence on science than even the federal granting system, say historians of science. The invasion of the university by corporations means that the objectivity of scientists is in question—more so than at any time in memory. Scientists who are tied to the biotech industry, those who have a monetary stake in it, can no longer claim to be disinterested. In evaluating what the technology can do and how much the nation needs it, their word is suspect. "It's the scientists who make the decisions about what the applications are and what risks are acceptable in light of the benefits," says Dutton. "But is that really what society as a whole would decide? I think the evidence indicates that the scientists' record is good in certain technical senses, but not nearly as good as it could be across a whole range of human values that make a society livable, and those are things lay people are expert on—truly expert."

Understanding Words in Context

Readers occasionally come across words which they do not recognize. And frequently, because they do not know a word or words, they will not fully understand the passage being read. Obviously, the reader can look up an unfamiliar word in a dictionary. However, by carefully examining the word in the context in which it is used, the word's meaning can often be determined. A careful reader may find clues to the meaning of the word in surrounding words, ideas, and attitudes.

Below are excerpts from the viewpoints in this chapter. In each excerpt, one or two words are printed in italics. Try to determine the meaning of each word by reading the excerpt. Under each excerpt you will find four definitions for the italicized word. Choose the one that is closest to your understanding of the word.

Finally, use a dictionary to see how well you have understood the words in context. It will be helpful to discuss with others the clues which helped you decide on each word's meaning.

1. Regulations must be appropriate, and should be based on consideration of the record of *NEGLIGIBLE* risk from genetic engineering to date, as well as on perceived risks and benefits.

   NEGLIGIBLE means:
   a) a very small amount   c) a large amount
   b) able to be changed   d) none at all

2. Suddenly gene technology, a subject that had been *RELEGATED* to the business section of the newspaper, was back on the front page.

   RELEGATED means:
   a) moved   c) left over from
   b) assigned more   d) assigned less
      importance   importance

3. What worries public interest groups most is the idea that biotechnology products, like those of other technologies, may *WREAK* changes that cannot be seen and perhaps not even measured.

WREAK means:
a) to destroy
b) to smell
c) to twist or pull
d) to cause

4. With computer programming of living systems, the very idea of nature being made up of *DISCRETE* species of living things, each with its own identity, becomes a thing of the past.

DISCRETE means:
a) distinct
b) unbelievable
c) cautious
d) camouflaged

5. A new ethics is being engineered, and its operating assumptions *COMPORT* nicely with the activity taking place in the biology laboratories.

COMPORT means:
a) play
b) agree
c) behave
d) add

6. Any resistance to the new technology will be *CASTIGATED* as inhuman, irresponsible, morally reprehensible and criminally liable.

CASTIGATED means:
a) punished
b) thrown out
c) criticized
d) listed

7. We remain apprentices to nature—and as *NOVICES* we must begin imitating her craft.

NOVICES means:
a) nuns
b) experts
c) young boys
d) beginners

8. A number of people in the scientific community drafted a letter asking that scientists not carry out certain kinds of experiments until experts could see whether they were safe. That produced a *MORATORIUM*.

MORATORIUM means:
a) a greenhouse
b) an agreement
c) a temporary ban
d) a monster

Periodical Bibliography

The following list of periodical articles deals with the subject matter of this chapter.

V. Elvig Anderson "Genetic Engineering: Is God's Image Endangered?" *Eternity,* November 1983.

Ronald Bailey "Fear and Loathing of Biotech's Bright Future," *Reason,* November 1985.

Dennis Chamberland "Genetic Engineering: Promise & Threat," *Christianity Today,* February 7, 1986.

Robert C. Cowen "Opening the Door to Progress in Genetic Engineering," *The Christian Science Monitor,* June 3, 1986.

Francis Crick "The Challenge of Biotechnology," *The Humanist,* July/August 1986.

Issues in Science and Technology "Genetic Engineering: Balancing Risk and Reward," Spring 1985. A series of three articles.

Horace Freeland Judson "Bioengineering and Ethics: Why Genetic Engineering?" *Current,* July/August 1985.

Jeff Lyon and Peter Gorner "Unlocking the Mysteries of DNA," *St. Paul Pioneer Press and Dispatch,* March 23, 1986.

Eliot Marshall "The Prophet Jeremy," *The New Republic,* December 10, 1984.

Kathleen McAuliffe and Sharon McAuliffe "Keeping Up with the Genetic Revolution," *The New York Times Magazine,* November 6, 1983.

Richard A. McCormick "Genetic Technology and Our Common Future," *America,* April 27, 1985.

Multinational Monitor Entire issue, February 28, 1986.

Richard Ness and Ruth Tonachel "Science May Bring Big Trouble for Farmers," *Minneapolis Star and Tribune,* July 6, 1986.

Keith Schneider "Weird Science," *Mother Jones,* November/December 1985.

Science 85 Several articles, November 1985.

Curtis J. Sitomer "Genetic Engineering," *The Christian Science Monitor,* September 25, 1986.

Are Organ Transplants Ethical?

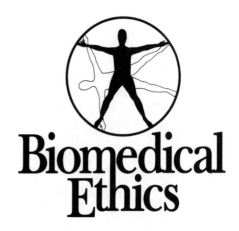

Biomedical Ethics

"Because of [organ transplants], many people are staying alive."

Organ Transplants Save Lives

Current Health 2

Millions of people have been the recipients of some type of organ transplant, whether the complicated and sometimes dangerous operation of a heart transplant or the more common process of a cornea transplant. The following viewpoint, taken from *Current Health 2* magazine, emphasizes the benefits of these transplants. The viewpoint stresses that, though not all transplants are successful, transplant technology has saved many lives. *Current Health 2* is a monthly magazine on health issues published for high school students.

As you read, consider the following questions:

1. According to the author, is organ transplant surgery cost effective?
2. What new technologies in transplants does the author describe?
3. What obstacle, according to the author, prevents patients from receiving organs they need?

"Organ Transplants: Ordinary Miracles, Extraordinary Results, *Current Health 2*, March 1986. Reprinted by permission.

The death of Pelle Lindbergh, a 26-year-old star hockey goalie in the prime of his career with the Philadelphia Flyers, devastated his family, his teammates, and his fans. But despite the sadness, Pelle's death and a courageous decision by his family touched the lives of several people who needed organ transplants.

Shortly after a car crash on an early Sunday morning [in] November [1985], doctors at a New Jersey hospital declared Pelle brain dead. Severe head injuries suffered in the accident gave him no chance of recovery; though his body continued to function with the help of a respirator, he had died. Realizing this, the Lindbergh family consented to donate Pelle's organs for transplantation. Most of the organs that can be used—kidneys, heart, liver, pancreas, corneas, skin, and bone—were recovered from Pelle's body and transplanted successfully. According to the agency that coordinated the recovery of the organs and the search for recipients, at least seven people were helped by the decision of Pelle Lindbergh's family.

Saving Lives

People like Pelle and his family have made a very special contribution to medical science—and to humanity. Because of their decision regarding organ donation, other people's lives will be saved. This is happening more frequently as technology and public awareness of the importance of organ donation increase. Some call organ transplants the gift of life; some call them ordinary miracles; others simply call them extraordinary. Whatever they are called, they now have become a vital part in the treatment of some disorders and diseases—and because of them, many people are staying alive. . . .

According to the Illinois Transplant Society, 200,000 people in the United States are waiting for transplants. More than 70,000 of them wait for vital organs such as a liver, heart, lung, kidney, or pancreas. Tissues including middle ear bone, bone marrow, the cornea of the eye, connective tissue, and skin also may be transplanted.

In 1984, 300 liver transplants, 225 heart transplants, 6,000 kidney transplants, and 24,000 cornea transplants were done. Liver replacement costs between $125,000 and $150,000. A healthy heart may cost as much as $100,000; a new kidney about $32,000. In financial terminology—is the surgery cost effective?

It costs $30,000 each year to maintain a person with kidney failure on dialysis (a kidney machine). A kidney transplant operation costs $30,000. But unlike a dialysis patient who remains very weak, most kidney transplant recipients recover completely and return to a normal life. Similarly, it costs $15,000 to rehabilitate a blind person; $3,000 for a cornea transplant. When the cause of blindness is a defective cornea, a cornea transplant can cure blindness.

Replacement organs are nothing short of a modern-day miracle. They both improve and extend lives. One year after surgery, more than 80 percent of those individuals who would have died without a donated organ are leading almost normal lives. . . .

Tricia

Each step Tricia took was painful. Even bending her knee joint was becoming more and more agonizing. Tricia's problem was that the *cartilage*, the gristle-like tissue that covered the tip of her lower leg bone, was wearing away. Finally, she consulted Dr. Marvin H. Meyers of the University of California-San Diego Medical School, who surgically treats many young people like Tricia who might otherwise require braces or fusion of the bones in their ailing joints.

Proven Effectiveness

Transplantation of human organs, primarily the kidney, heart, and liver, has become an effective means of treating many patients who have life-threatening organ failure. Organ transplantation is now widely available in this country and of proven effectiveness.

Department of Health and Human Services, *Report of the Task Force on Organ Transplantation,* April 1986.

For Tricia's operation, Dr. Meyers first removed the dead cartilage. He then replaced it with a composite graft, a portion of donated bone with cartilage on top of it. Dr. Meyers had to measure and cut the composite graft so it would fit and inlay it by pressing it into place on Tricia's bone.

Dr. Meyers has performed similar operations on shattered hips and ankles. These operations can help prevent deformity due to injury, but, Dr. Meyers cautions, are not useful in restoring joints damaged by arthritis. Though cartilage is an "immunologically privileged tissue," that is, not attacked by the immune system, Dr. Meyers claims that a cartilage transplant cannot replace a joint damaged by rheumatoid arthritis because the disease process would destroy the replaced cartilage as well. However, some osteoarthritis patients and Tricia, whose problem was not arthritis but a lack of blood circulation in her knee, could walk again without pain after a bone and cartilage transplant.

Since some physicians repair damaged bones with segments of fibula, the smaller bone in the lower leg, both bone and cartilage banks would greatly benefit those with bone injuries or disease.

Transplants can also be hearing aids. How? By replacing damaged bones in the ear.

Injury or infection can damage the eardrum or the three small bones of the middle ear. This causes a *conductive hearing loss,* to which sound is not amplified. To restore the eardrum, Dr. Arvind Kumar, associate professor and director of neurotology, University of Illinois Medical Center, Chicago, uses *fascia,* or connective tissue, covering one of the muscles above the patient's ear. Middle ear bones are taken from a bone bank where they can be stored for as long as a year. No tissue matching is required since rejection is not a problem. Says Dr. Kumar, "With proper care and measurements, transplanted fascia and middle ear bones can fully restore hearing.". . .

Leg Transplants

What's the next human body part that will be replaced? Look to the latest animal transplants. All transplants are done on animals before they are done on humans. Recently, researchers at the University of California-Irvine transplanted legs onto laboratory rats. The transplanted legs survived throughout the rats' three-year lifespan. Several of the animals did not reject the new limbs, even when the immune-suppressant drug cyclosporin was discontinued.

What makes these transplanted legs so revolutionary is that they are transplants of composite tissue—containing skin, muscle, bone, blood vessels, and nerves. The transplant involves *microsurgery,* surgery done while looking through a microscope, to reattach tiny structures such as nerves and blood vessels. Because the rats' new legs exhibited near-normal muscle and nerve activity, researchers think that composite grafts might replace artificial limbs or treat massive tissue destruction in humans.

If limbs . . . can be transplanted, what's next? Researchers are looking into the possibility of brain implants or brain tissue grafts. Because the brain is the seat of emotions, intellect, and personality, most people object to the idea of brain transplants. Nevertheless, brain researchers are pinpointing areas of the brain involved in functions such as movement, sensation, and memory. In the 21st century, will brain implants cure paralysis, blindness, or memory loss?

Transplantation is a rapidly improving therapy. Only 20 years ago, most people who received transplanted organs died. Today, new surgical techniques and immunosuppressive drugs allow transplant patients to lead normal lives.

"The cadaver has come to have a market value, leaving no place for requiems, prayers, or mourning."

Organ Transplants Are Destroying Human Values

Malcolm Muggeridge

Organ transplants have been a part of medical technology for many decades and have prolonged many lives. Not all observers are convinced of their benefit to humanity, however. In the following viewpoint, Malcolm Muggeridge voices his fear that organ transplants are eroding the values that have upheld Western civilization for centuries. Muggeridge, the well-known editor of *Punch*, a British humor magazine, has written numerous books and achieved world fame as a lecturer and broadcaster.

As you read, consider the following questions:

1. According to Muggeridge, what part of human beings is modern medicine ignoring?
2. The author uses an argument called "the slippery slope," which says that small moral concessions will lead to total abandonment of ethical principles. How does he relate this argument to organ transplants?

Malcolm Muggeridge, "Medical Progress and the Human Soul," *The Human Life Review*, April 1986. Reprinted with the author's permission.

The whole apparatus of medicine has achieved the most fantastic results in recent years. Nobody can possibly deny that. Illnesses which in my childhood were household words have disappeared; for instance, illnesses like diphtheria. Those who have achieved all this are to be greatly thanked. At the same time, we have to realize—at least, I *think* we have to realize—that whereas in abolishing these illnesses, doctors have achieved great things with human flesh, they have not achieved anything much for the human soul. Has not the human soul, in fact, tended to wither away because of the attention given, almost exclusively (and with fine results) to the body?

This is the basic question that I have tried to look at; the more I look at it, however, the more complicated it becomes.

I also had a feeling about it all which was personal and perhaps rather egotistic; but as I read about the amazing achievements made by transplanting organs, I could not help reflecting that a rather charming little poem of Byron's, which I had cherished, would no longer be singable in our world. The poem, addressed to the Maid of Athens, begins like this:

> Maid of Athens, ere we part
> Give, O give me back my heart!
> But since that has left my breast,
> Take, O take, O take the rest!

Now that is a charming little love song, but who will be able to sing it without indulging in the kind of ribaldry with which it has been received here? . . .

A Growing Traffic in Organs

In the field of transplant surgery there is another problem: the growing traffic in organs. Putting them on the market is becoming an extraordinarily lucrative occupation. There was a newspaper report recently telling us that you could get a lot of dollars for a kidney in good condition. That is going to be a very big trade and, furthermore, of course, you could carry it further and go in for mass commerce of various parts of the body. They have not yet had any testicles on the market, but I daresay they will have a very good price, too, if they do get on the market; probably better than kidneys! It is a matter of opinion, I suppose.

There is, no doubt, a big demand for organs for transplantation, but, to an old fellow like me, it all has an unsavory feeling about it: you are taking from cadavers or from living human beings, organs they are prepared to get rid of, or, as is tragically the case, from people in the world who are so poor, so without the necessities of life, that they are prepared to offer their own organs for sale in order to be able to satisfy themselves in other directions. Now to me, at any rate, this is a sort of very sad thing. One cannot actually nail down why it seems horrible that a kidney should be sold for a large sum of money, or that there are people so desperately in need of kidneys that they are prepared to pay large sums for them, but to me these contracts have something very creepy and unpleasant about them. This may be just prejudice, and it may be that when I have departed this world, which will be quite soon, and had some rest in a better place (I hope),

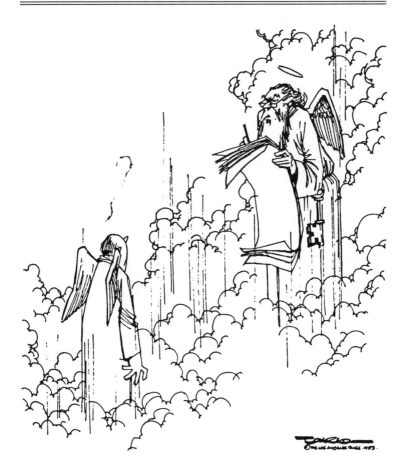

"BARNEY CLARK...YOU'RE 112 DAYS LATE!"

I shall see that it's all to the good. But I feel in my bones that there is something terrible in it.

We are in danger, it seems to me, of losing the respect for the dead which has prevailed through the centuries, not just of Christendom, but of other civilizations as well. The practice has been to cover dead bodies respectfully, recognizing that, with the departure of the soul, the remainder is just a carcass to be disposed of by burial or cremation. Now, however, there is the possibility of financial deals with dead bodies; the cadaver has come to have a market value, leaving no place for requiems, prayers, or mourning with kidneys, hearts, eyeballs and other such items up for sale.

The Breakdown of Civilization

You can speak of strict controls, but when it comes to the point in matters of this kind, controls go by the board. When the abortion bill was being canvassed, the argument all the time was, "Of course we don't want people to have abortions, of course we're going to have the best possible means of dealing with that, but it must be available for us." And yet, within a matter of months or even weeks, those who had brought in the bill were complaining that they had no idea it would result in the current absolute holocaust. At the present moment, it is believed with reason that in England a human fetus is being disposed of every three minutes. These things are happening, and they are happening not because those concerned in the mechanism of the bill are heartless or brutal, but because it places us on a slippery slope. In the case of abortion, one can see that, once you accept its validity, then the slippery slope works. So, in the end, you finish up with the strange, and, I think, terrifying situation which you have today of abortion being done incessantly, on the one hand, and of underage children being encouraged to receive contraceptives, on the other.

All these things, which will be in the history books, are marking the total decadence, the breakdown, of what is called Western Civilization. I believe that the people who are working even in the field of transplantation, in the most respectful way, and believing that what they are doing is good, should think very carefully about what the consequences of that sort of thing can be if it gets out of control.

"Our culture works awfully hard to avoid the taint of money in organ donations: the gift of life must always remain a gift."

Purchasing Organs Is Unethical

Thomas H. Murray

Due to a shortage of organ donors, many patients with weak or damaged organs wait for months for transplants. Some die before a donor can be found. In the following viewpoint, Thomas H. Murray discusses how this organ shortage can be eliminated. Though he acknowledges the temptation to treat the human body as property, he believes organs should always be donated as gifts, never sold for profit. Murray teaches ethics at the University of Texas Medical School in Galveston, Texas.

As you read, consider the following questions:

1. Why is the John Moore case important to Murray's discussion of donating organs?
2. What three possible models does Murray offer for thinking about attitudes toward organ donation?
3. According to the author, why is the removal of an organ, such as a kidney, fundamentally different from having one's blood drawn or hair cut?

Thomas H. Murray, "The Gift of Life Must Always Remain a Gift," *Discover*, March 1986. © *Discover* Magazine. Reprinted by permission.

The call came early in the morning. It was a staffer from a congressional subcommittee. The chairman had become interested in the issues raised by the Mo Cell case. Would I come to Washington and testify?

My first reaction was to laugh. I knew the case. John Moore had been a cancer patient with hairy-cell leukemia. There was no treatment for it except to remove his dangerously enlarged spleen. So they had plucked it out, and some scientists at UCLA had managed to grow Moore's cells—labeled Mo for short—in the laboratory; an immortal cell line, they called it, because, unlike most cells from mammals, Moore's cancerous spleen cells didn't stop replicating after a few dozen divisions. None of that was so new; immortal cell lines have contributed vastly to medical research. What made the case noteworthy was that UCLA and the scientists patented the Mo line—and then John Moore sued them.

The Mo cell seemed to belong in the Mondo Ethico category—a name coined by a friend and me for bizarre cases in bioethics. That was why I laughed. But when Congress calls, the least you owe them is to think it over. So I said I would brood about it, and talk to them later in the day.

Provocative Questions

Once I began to think about the case, though, it obsessed me. The questions were so provocative: What is our relationship with diseased parts of our bodies once they have been removed? Do scientists have any right to get rich from our misfortune? Are there any good analogies for thinking about these issues?

Such questions wouldn't have been raised ten or twenty years ago, before biotechnology captured the imagination of the American public—and Wall Street. No one worried about winning any biotechnology lottery, because there was nothing to win. Like most basic researchers, biologists labored in relative anonymity and poverty. Yet with the sudden blossoming of genetic engineering, monoclonal antibodies, and other technologies, biologists have found that the distance from the lab to the condo in St. Moritz isn't so far.

However, the birth of biotechnology only explains why the question of who should profit from human cell lines hasn't arisen before now. While modern biology's age of innocence may have passed, we must still decide how it should behave as a responsible adult. The Mo Cell case may be one of its severest tests.

The first thing I realized about this case was that we needed models for thinking about our relationship with our body parts once they were no longer joined with the living whole. There seemed to be three possibilities: the body as property, as surplus, and as a gift.

The Body as Property

If the body is property, then it can be bought and sold like other commodities. The only question in the Mo Cell case then would be who owns it *now?* Did Moore abandon or transfer title to his spleen cells when he let UCLA remove them?

There are reasons for thinking of the body as property. We allow the sale of such things as hair, sperm, and blood. But these are all replenishable (usually), and that may be the vital difference. Also, those of us who work at hazardous occupations risk our bodies, or at least our health, for money every workday. But risking our health isn't really the same thing as selling our bodies. Imagine someone making a living by betting his pancreas against someone else's cash. Even if the odds were awfully good, I suspect we would see that as wrong. It's one thing to risk our health at work, quite another to wager our bodies.

Voluntary Giving

Moral wisdom lies, we believe, in the position taken by the Uniform Anatomical Gift Act. It is true that the emphasis on voluntary giving rather than on routine taking of organs may well insure a perpetual shortage of cadaver organs. And this is morally serious. On the other hand, the rule of organized, voluntary giving seems to recognize the danger in our developing a "spare-parts" mentality about our bodies. It recognizes the problems that would be faced in their hours of grief by families who feel deeply about the body remaining intact and yet who would have to resist routine hospital procedures. It recognizes that however great the need for transplant organs, we need to be at least as concerned about how those organs are obtained. And it recognizes that in matters as personal as this, society will be better served if it can rely on voluntary giving rather than on routine taking.

James B. Nelson and Jo Anne Smith Rohricht, *Human Medicine: Ethical Perspectives on Today's Medical Issues*, 1984.

In fact, there are better reasons for thinking that we don't regard the body as commercial property. Even in the culture that spawned *Let's Make a Deal*, not everything is for sale. We aren't permitted to sell our freedom, our children, or, most recently, our transplantable organs— though the shortage of human organs has led to a couple of lamentable efforts. In one case, ads appeared in the classified sections of newspapers offering kidneys for sale. (We have two kidneys, but can live with just one). In another, a man tried to peddle his liver, until it was pointed out to him that we're not born with spares. A Virginia physician, who had set himself up as a broker in human organs, went so far as to procure a license to import organs from overseas.

A Ban on Selling Organs

This was too much for Congress, which in 1984 passed a bill banning the buying or selling of organs for transplant. (People just don't take kindly to the thought of an organ mogul sipping champagne next to his kidney-or heart-shaped swimming pool.)

Why the moral repugnance toward trading in human organs? One reason may be fear of the development of a market in which the poor do the selling and the rich the buying. Our consciences can tolerate considerable injustice, but such naked, undisguised profiteering in life would be too much for most of us.

And even if everyone had an equal chance to buy and sell, I doubt that we'd countenance a market in human organs. The notion that people are special, that they have a dignity and moral worth that sets them apart, is deeply woven into our religious, legal, and political traditions. We may be more than mere protoplasm, but we're nothing without our bodies (at least in this world). Putting a price on the priceless, even a high price, actually cheapens it. So we don't approve of selling our body parts; and the body isn't quite property. . . .

The Body as Gift

A physician friend once told me of a young boy with a rare blood deficiency. His blood lacked one of the factors that enables it to clot, though not the one (Factor VIII) whose absence commonly causes hemophilia. The blood's unusual properties made it exceedingly valuable to medical researchers, and for about a year the boy came regularly to the medical center to donate blood for research. Then a pharmaceutical company learned of the youngster, and hit upon a way to use his blood profitably. They asked him for it and he agreed to give it—for a stiff price. The same blood that had been donated to the scientists suddenly became a commodity. The boy and his family apparently felt that it was right, even noble, to give the blood without remuneration to the scientists. With equal conviction, they also apparently believed that it would be foolish to make a gift of it to a company that planned to sell it to make money.

This story tells us that people regard their relationships with scientific researchers as drastically different from their relationships with profit-seeking corporations. Scientists are engaged in a socially valued enterprise in which they aren't expected to grow wealthy; corporations exist to maximize their wealth. We can have a relationship with scientists based on gifts; nobody has a gift relationship with General Dynamics (except perhaps the Pentagon).

Nothing more clearly illuminates the gift nature of transactions involving our organs than the "gift of life" itself—donating organs for transplantation. Most organs come from cadavers, although roughly a third of the kidneys come from live donors, almost always close kin of the recipients. The model law authorizing organ donation is called the Uniform Anatomical *Gift* Act. The organ banks responsible for procuring organs go to great lengths to make certain that while the donors or their heirs aren't financially penalized for their generosity, neither are they given monetary inducements. The itemized hospital bill is carefully examined; only those charges relating to the organ donation are paid by the organ bank. Our culture works awfully hard to avoid the taint of money in organ donations: the gift of life must always remain a gift. . . .

An Economic Argument

Besides the moral arguments against an organ market, there is an economic one: that it might well raise the cost of organs without doing much to increase the supply. People who now donate organs for altruistic reasons might demand payment instead, or, convinced that the market was taking care of things, they might decline to part with their organs at all. The elasticity of supply and demand may not apply in the emotionally charged atmosphere of a hospital waiting room, where the next of kin are considering how to dispose of Mom.

Bill Keller, *The New Republic*, March 19, 1984.

The real danger from the Mo Cell case and others that may follow is that they threaten to transform the nature of the relationship between scientists and the public. People have been generous with science, especially in making gifts of themselves in the form of tissues and organs. If they begin to see scientists as greedy players in a biotechnology lottery with tickets provided by public generosity, this relationship stands to change, and not for the better.

Whether or not John Moore wins his suit isn't the fundamental issue. His case will probably be decided more by the vagaries of the patent laws than by any ethical analysis. At the heart of the matter is whether the gift relationship between science and the public can continue, or whether *caveat donor* becomes the new rule. Scientists are going to have to face this issue squarely. If public trust, esteem, and generosity are important to them, then a little generosity in turn is a small price to pay for sustaining a mutually satisfying relationship. Otherwise, this could be the beginning of the end of a beautiful friendship.

"Just as oilmen need incentives to drill, people need incentives to donate organs."

Purchasing Organs Is Practical

Fern Schumer Chapman, Emanuel Thorne and Gilah Langner

Fern Schumer Chapman, a free-lance writer, held the 1984-85 Ivan F. Boesky fellowship for journalists at the Harvard School of Public Health. Emanuel Thorne and Gilah Langner are economic consultants who have studied the use of human biological material for research and commerce. In Part I of the following viewpoint, Chapman suggests forming a commercial market for cadaver organs. In Part II, Thorne and Langner advocate the same idea. All three authors argue that economic incentives will eliminate the organ shortage and provide transplants to all who need them.

As you read, consider the following questions:

1. According to Chapman, what are the less desirable alternatives to an organ market?
2. How has the value of the human body changed, according to Thorne and Langner?
3. Chapman, Thorne, and Langner believe donors should be paid. Do you agree? Why or why not?

I

There are some problems the government simply can't solve. And often the government only makes matters worse. The USA's vital organ shortage is one of those problems.

At issue is how to increase organ donations. A federal task force is recommending that states pass legislation requiring hospitals to ask relatives of all suitable patients for organs and that the federal government organize a network to match donors and recipients.

No Incentives

All this may help, but it doesn't address the root of the problem: There are no incentives to induce organ donations beyond a donor's selfless impulse. The USA would be a utopia if all of its citizens had that selfless impulse. But, unfortunately, they don't. And it's unrealistic for the government to expect that kind of altruism.

There is a simple solution to the problem—a commercial market in cadaver organs. However, the government has already foreclosed that option. A . . . federal law explicitly bans the buying and selling of live or cadaver organs and carries a $50,000 fine or a prison term as long as five years.

But the numbers make the best case for a market.

Each year, organs are taken from only 3,500 of the nation's 20,000 potential donors—otherwise healthy people who suffer brain deaths in a hospital. In addition, there is a shocking waste of organs, an estimated 20 percent of all those donated. A market would not only increase the supply but eliminate the waste.

The choice is simple—an organ and a price or no organ and no price. Society doesn't expect people to work for free. So why does it expect people to give organs for nothing?

In a cadaver market, donors could contract with a firm to sell their usable body parts upon their death, with a fee to be paid to their estates. Or, a health insurance agency could pay the closest living relative for his dead relative's organs.

The people of the USA could tolerate a market sooner than some of the alternatives such as European-style "presumed consent" laws under which the state assumes that it can harvest the organs of anyone who dies in a hospital. We here are sure to resist this noting of nationalized corpses.

People in the USA would like medicine to operate on some high plane, beyond the considerations of profit and price. It seems ghoulish to put a price on an organ, or, even worse, a life. But medicine is a market like any other, and functions by the same principles as, say, the oil market.

Just as oilmen need incentives to drill, people need incentives to donate organs. In either case, when there are none, a shortage develops. With organs, the stakes are incomparably higher: life or death for thousands.

Organ donations are too important to be left to the whims of altruism or the dead weight of government bureaucracy.

II

Until recently, it was possible to joke that the value of the body, based on its chemical constituents, was about $1.98. Now, its value exceeds $200,000 and is rising. Tissue is being harvested for transplantation, research and diagnostic and therapeutic products. In 1985, nearly 8,000 kidneys and 20,000 corneas were transplanted; heart transplants are being performed at the rate of 1,200 per year.

Market Proposals

If something doesn't happen to get the present [voluntary] system off the dime, we're going to hear about strong market proposals in the near future. . . .

Remember, you can sell plasma in the United States. Sperm donors are routinely reimbursed. And surrogate mothers are often paid to rent their wombs.

Arthur Caplan, in *Mother Jones*, December 1984.

The value of tissue created by the revolution in biotechnology raises anew important ethical, legal and economic issues involving how this value is to be shared. In a case in California, for example, a former leukemia patient is suing for the value of his spleen, which was removed during his treatment and used to develop a patentable product subsequently licensed to a biotechnology company.

The 1984 National Organ Transplantation Act prohibited sales of organs for transplantation, reflecting Congressional concern for individual and public health and for the nation's moral sensitivity. The ethical position embodied in the prohibition of "organ markets," however, seems to ignore economic realities that may undermine Congressional intent. A law prohibiting sales of organs does not make them valueless. Such a law only bars organ suppliers from reaping the economic value of their organs. The law makes organs free goods that can be harvested by anyone who can establish a claim to them.

To understand how the intent of the 1984 law might be subverted, imagine that a market for transplantable kidneys exists. Say there are three parties to a transaction: a donor, a surgical-and-hospital team and the recipient, and they are able to carry out all the transaction at prices agreeable to all. Let's assume that the amount required by the owner of the kidney to provide the kidney is $20,000, the amount for the team's services is $30,000 and the recipient is willing to pay the total sum of $50,000.

Suppose that a law like the 1984 act is passed requiring all transplants to be gifts. Who would reap the $20,000 value of the kidney? Undoubtedly, the intent of the law was to treat the kidney as a gift to the recipient; thus, he pays $30,000 rather than $50,000. However, nothing in the law insures this outcome. The medical team could reap the entire value of the kidney by charging the recipient $50,000.

Transplants for Foreigners

A series of articles in *The Pittsburgh Press* in 1985 reported that in 1984-85, while nationwide 10,000 Americans waited for transplants, at several hospitals nearly 30 percent of kidney transplants were performed on foreigners allowed to jump the queue of Americans, and that surgeons' fees were as much as four times and hospital charges almost twice as high for foreigners as for Americans. The Department of Health and Human Services confirmed . . . that a high percentage of American kidneys were being transplanted into foreigners who were being charged fees several times that charged Americans.

Is that what Congress had in mind in passing the law? No. Nor is it what most organ donors and their families have in mind. Potential donors may be happy donating to sick foreigners but not if those foreigners are given an unfair advantage over equally needy Americans. . . .

A Federal task force on transplantation recently called for important changes in the system, including creation of a nationwide organ procurement system, Government financing of transplants for the poor and a limit of transplants into foreigners of 10 percent of kidneys from cadavers. Even these steps will not eliminate financial and distributional inequities if the system leaves the values of the organ up for grabs.

However repugnant the idea, the body now has economic value that cannot be wished away or ignored. As new techniques increase the value of the body, the nation will need far more stringent controls in order to preserve the trust between donors and recipients. But if we are unwilling or unable to organize an efficient and equitable system in which the generosity of donors is not abused, then it may be time to consider paying donors for their organs.

"People could be saved if the artificial-heart program were given the fast experimental track."

The Artificial Heart Should Be Used

Harry Schwartz

In December 1982 a dentist from Seattle named Barney Clark became the first recipient of an artificial heart. He subsequently lived for 112 days. In the following viewpoint, Harry Schwartz chastises those who, since Barney Clark's death, have held back the artificial-heart program. No expense should be spared, he says, in implementing a device that could save so many lives. Schwartz, formerly a member of the Editorial Board of *The New York Times*, is writer in residence at the College of Physicians and Surgeons at Columbia University.

As you read, consider the following questions:

1. According to Schwartz, what caused Dr. William C. DeVries, the surgeon who implanted an artificial heart in Barney Clark, to leave the University of Utah heart program?
2. What, according to Schwartz, is the basic advantage of an artificial heart?

Harry Schwartz, "Cut the Red Tape; Implant at Full Speed," *The New York Times*, August 17, 1984. Copyright © 1984 by The New York Times Company. Reprinted by permission.

Congress should hold public hearings on the barriers that . . . have prevented further experiments involving implanting artificial hearts in humans.

The artificial heart is probably the most important recent medical advance on which experimentation has begun. Yet an absurd mass of red tape and the thinly hidden fears of business and Government leaders who would rather save dollars than save lives have so frustrated Barney Clark's surgeon, Dr. William C. DeVries, that he has left the University of Utah to join the Humana Heart Institute, a part of the Humana Corporation, a private hospital chain based in Louisville, Ky.

Sabotage

Even while Barney Clark lived, those who fear the cost implications of a successful artificial heart were trying to sabotage Dr. DeVries's work. In January 1983, six weeks into Mr. Clark's life with the artificial heart, I went to Salt Lake City to research an article on the implant. I interviewed, among others, Dr. Willem Kolff, the inventor of kidney dialysis and the leader of the team that produced the Jarvik-7 artificial heart, named for its designer, Dr. Robert Jarvik. Dr. Kolff told me then that a leading Utah medical figure had appealed to the state's Governor, Scott M. Matheson, to order the plug pulled on—that is, to kill—Barney Clark. The reason? It was feared that the expense of maintaining Mr. Clark (the total bill came to more than $250,000) on the artificial heart was too great. Since then it has been obvious that in Washington and in Utah there are powerful opponents of further human experimentation with the artificial heart. The Food and Drug Administration took more than a year to grant permission for a second human trial, and the University of Utah committee on human experimentation, a peer review group, was similarly dilatory.

Historically, the Federal Government has supported most American medical research, but it is clearly becoming tired of paying the bills. Humana has pledged to pay millions of dollars for up to 100 artificial heart operations, operations for which the University of Utah had no funds. Humana is taking a substantial risk, but if this research succeeds humanity will be the winner.

One need not be a great medical specialist to understand that Barney Clark's experience was a triumph for humanity and for the device's makers. That Mr. Clark survived at all after receiving the artificial heart is a minor miracle, for he was almost dead when the new heart was implanted in his chest. Once minutes from death, he was kept alive for four months and recovered enough to conduct his historic televised conversation with Dr. DeVries.

Some critics have complained that Mr. Clark obviously had a hard time during the months a pump propelled his blood. But would he have been better off dead? And isn't it reasonable to suppose that if he had gotten the new heart when he was in better shape, he would have had a fuller and more rapid recovery? . . .

Technology Advances

I believe it is necessary to make clear where I stand in regard to the artificial heart. There is no question that the amount of money being used to produce and implant the artificial heart could improve the health of many more individuals if it were employed for preventive services. But that, and many other objections that are raised against the advance of high technology are, to me, beside the point. Technology advances whether one agrees or not. One can turn aside or join, but as has been frequently noted, technology has its own imperative. Personally, I enjoy it.

Eric J. Cassell, in *After Barney Clark*, 1984.

In my research, I was shocked to discover that some heart-transplant surgeons were doing their best to badmouth Dr. DeVries's work and the artificial heart. Their fear that heart transplants might be made obsolete by a successful artificial heart was very evident. Yet the basic advantage of an artificial heart is that, unlike natural hearts, it can be manufactured in any quantity desired.

Dr. DeVries's frustrating experience has also highlighted the cumbersomeness of the whole complicated program for getting permission to do such experiments. Few medical events in the modern world have been so minutely publicized and scrutinized as the experiment to which Barney Clark gave himself. But that did not prevent the bureaucratic nightmare that finally forced Dr. DeVries to leave Utah.

Every day thousands of people die of heart ailments, the biggest killer of Americans. Some, perhaps many, of these people could be saved if the artificial-heart program were given the fast experimental track.

Perhaps our society can't afford to give an artificial heart to every person who needs one. If so, we can decide later how to ration these organs. Meanwhile, Congress ought to investigate those who have been sabotaging this program and do whatever is needed to permit it to go ahead at full speed.

"It is time for a moratorium on the implantation of artificial hearts."

The Artificial Heart Should Not Be Used

B.D. Colen

B.D. Colen, science editor of *Newsday*, won the 1985 Page One Award for Science Reporting. He has written several books including *Hard Choices: Mixed Blessings of Modern Medical Technology* from which this viewpoint is taken. Colen calls the artificial-heart program a failure. He believes the artificial heart is not only unethical, but too expensive. It should be sent back to the lab for more experimentation, he states, while congressional committees examine the current state of natural and artificial organ transplantation.

As you read, consider the following questions:

1. What, according to Colen, is the artificial-heart program doing to the rest of the health care system?
2. What examples does Colen give of the program's failure?
3. Do you agree with Colen that the artificial heart is too expensive? Why or why not?

After thirty-one years of kidney transplantation and eighteen years of transplanting human hearts, we still have not worked out a uniform process either to select patients for these procedures or to pay for them. We have not, in fact, even figured out if we should be providing them. As George Annas asks, "Should we be doing these transplants at all? Are these procedures so expensive that until we have some system to ensure that everyone in America has a basic minimum of health care we shouldn't be adding these extremely expensive halfway technologies? It skews the system. One of my colleagues says aptly: 'We have been doing more and more to fewer and fewer people at higher and higher cost for less and less benefit.' We are getting more and more people who are being completely cut out of the system. Thirty-five million Americans do not have insurance. Most are under twenty-four years old. We are doing more and more medicine to people at the later end of life. When you add something," Annas notes, "you take something away. It's a tradeoff system."

A Failure

What are the tradeoffs involved in the quickly burgeoning artificial-heart program? As of 1985, the open-minded can only call this initial program a failure. Barney Clark, the Seattle dentist who served as the first human guinea pig for Dr. William DeVries and his team at the University of Utah, was described to and in the media as a pioneer, a brave explorer of medical frontiers who, in the hopes his life would be extended, agreed to be the first human in whom a Jarvik-7 polyurethane and alloy heart would be implanted. But did Clark have the vaguest idea what he was getting into when he made that agreement? While he may not have honestly believed he would ever go home to Seattle, did he think he would spend his "extra" 112 days in the hospital, slowly deteriorating as his physicians helped him from one medical crisis to the next? Could he have had any way to anticipate a second open-heart procedure to replace a broken—untested— valve in the artificial heart? Could he have anticipated such severe and repeated nosebleeds that he required surgery to stop them? Could he, or should his surgeons, have anticipated an incapacitating stroke—caused by a blood clot formed as a direct result of the artificial heart's use—that would leave him little more than a vegetable? Is that what Barney Clark opted for when he agreed to surgery at the University of Utah?

And what of William Schroeder, the "tough," "spunky" former federal employee and union leader who underwent the same procedure, seemed to be recovering beautifully and then suffered a stroke just as Clark had. We were told he was doing better, but then when the shell of a man was brought before television cameras it was painfully obvious he barely seemed to know who or where he was, or what was going on. Then a great todo was made—by hospital officials and the media—over the fact that Schroeder was leaving the hospital and "going home." But "home" was a special apartment, a specially equipped hospital room, really, less than 120 seconds away from the specialists in the hospital across the street. Then Schroeder suffered yet another stroke and was back in the hospital—where he suffered a third, major stroke. Yes, as of the end of 1985 Schroeder had "survived" for more than a year. But the William Schroeder who survived scarcely resembled the William Schroeder whom surgeon DeVries operated on. Is this the kind of survival Schroeder and his family had in mind when he agreed to the implant?

A Handful of Artificial Hearts

Even assuming that artificial hearts can be developed that will work well through the normal life span of a patient, how many tens or hundreds of thousands of dollars are justified in a single case of life saving? . . .

Those of us who have waded through the dismal swamps of endemic poverty in much of the world see where the cost of a handful of heart transplants could save the sight, vigor and even the lives of thousands.

Jenkin Lloyd Jones, *Conservative Chronicle*, September 10, 1986.

And what of Murray Haydon? As someone callously but quite aptly described the situation when the Humana Heart Institute International announced that an operation to implant a heart in Haydon had gone "perfectly" and he was bouncing right back, it reminded one of the family who has a dying old dog and goes out and buys a new puppy to distract the children from the death of their beloved pet. Not only did Humana attempt to switch media attention from Schroeder to Haydon, but reporters—and Schroeder's family members—were not even told how bad things looked for Schroeder until *after* the fanfare for the success of the Haydon procedure. And look what happened to Haydon: a second surgical procedure and then "life"—dependent upon a respirator. The next patient, Jack Burcham, died only ten days after receiving the artificial heart. DeVries at least finally acknowledged in an interview that the procedure is experimental, rather than therapeutic. But Robert Jarvik, the inventor of the heart, told *Newsday* medical writer David Zinman that he believes stroke is an acceptable complication to the use of an artificial heart. "Life with

87

stroke is better than death and [is] an acceptable quality of life," said the physician-inventor, who himself has never experienced life either with stroke or with his invention. . . .

Unauthorized Experiments

[Thomas] Creighton, a thirty-three-year-old mechanic, was dying of heart disease when surgeons at the University of Arizona gave him a heart transplant. All well and good. But the new human heart was rejected, and so the doctors called for an artificial heart—which they were not authorized to implant. Rather than wait an extra two hours for a Jarvik-7, which has at least been extensively tested on animals and has been cleared by the FDA [Food and Drug Administration] for human implantation, the Tucson surgeons gave Creighton a heart designed by a dentist and, essentially, never tested. (In a discussion of artificial hearts, twelve hours of testing is tantamount to never being tested.) Then, less than twelve hours after Creighton was given the implant, the surgeons removed it and he underwent a second human heart transplant. That operation, like the first, was a failure, and Creighton died forty-six hours after first being placed on the surgical merry-go-round.

The surgeons justified their action by, one, saying that Creighton would have died without the implant, as though patients don't die every day, and two, saying that doctors answer to a higher power than the FDA. The FDA responded to this clear violation of federal regulation by investigating and then failing to take any action aganst the surgeon involved. In fact, it later gave him place number three on the list of surgeons approved to implant Jarvik-7's. What message does this send to other doctors who want to carry on their own experiments, using the justification that the patient is dying? What may ultimately be even more disturbing is the fact that the surgeon, Jack Copeland, said he will be using the Jarvik-7 as a bridge to human transplantation in cases where a patient needs a human heart transplant but there is no organ available. Copeland said he views the Jarvik-7 as just "another modality" available to save lives—although at the time it had only been used on five patients and had triggered strokes in four of those.

Can We Afford It?

Even if these problems were not arising, if doctors were not becoming more inclined to experiment on helpless, dying patients, if there were no ethical, legal, bureaucratic or even public relations problems here, we are still left with the question of whether we can afford an artificial-heart program that will cost more than the entire gross national product of many semideveloped nations. It is now estimated that anywhere from 10,000 to 60,000 persons would be candidates each year for an artificial heart implant.

Assume there are 50,000. And assume the procedure and attendant treatment will cost *only* $100,000 per patient. That's $5 billion (not million) a year for this one medical procedure. In other words, we would be spending more than twice what we are now spending on kidney dialysis and we will be spending it not to give a new life to children or young adults, but to persons on the verge of retirement, individuals who are likely to develop other diseases and complications in a relatively short period.

Assume, for a moment, that such a program makes social, if not financial sense. After all, the people receiving these hearts have—at least as a group—contributed to society all their lives and it can be easily argued that they are then entitled to society's support in return. However, once they have been given an artificial heart, what happens when that heart gives out? Bioethicist Robert Veatch makes the interesting argument that, while society does not have an obligation to provide an artificial heart in the first place, it *does* have an obligation to replace that heart when it breaks down. And like refrigerators, artificial hearts will give out, probably in five years or less. Assuming that most individuals receive their first

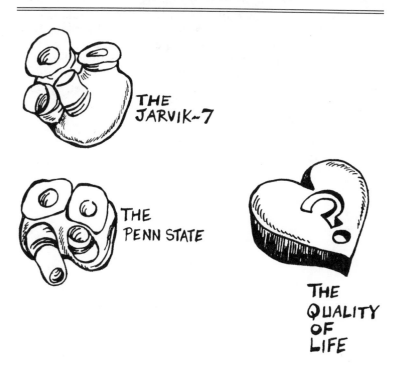

THE
JARVIK-7

THE
PENN STATE

THE
QUALITY
OF
LIFE

© Boileau/Rothco

artificial heart at age fifty-five and live another twenty years, we could be talking about supplying each individual with not one but *four* artificial hearts. Or we could be talking about spending not $100,000 per patient but $400,000 per patient, or $20 billion a year.

Time for a Moratorium

Clearly, then, it is time for a moratorium on the implantation of artificial hearts. This device may eventually prove to be an enormous boon to mankind. It may save 50,000 lives a year. It may be worth the billions that would be required to make it available. But first we should consider the proper place the device might have in the overall treatment of heart disease after it has been sent back to the animal lab for refinement. The most sensible course of action at this time would be for one of the congressional appropriation committees to establish a national organ transplantation commission to examine the current state of organ transplantation, both natural and artificial. Such a commission should examine the medical, ethical and financial questions at the heart of the transplantation efforts and, as society's representative, make the hard choices that must be made. Should such a commission come down against public funding of organ transplantation, it should decide whether transplants should be available at all. And if it decides that transplants should be publicly funded, the commission should decide what programs will be eliminated to provide the billions of dollars needed to finance a universal organ transplantation program. And, finally, Congress must then be willing to act on the commission's recommendations.

Distinguishing Between Fact and Opinion

This activity is designed to help develop the basic critical thinking skill of distinguishing between fact and opinion. Consider the following statement as an example: "According to the Illinois Transplant Society, 200,000 people in the United States are waiting for transplants." This statement is a fact with which no one who has looked at the research could disagree. But consider another statement about organ transplants: "Organ transplants are worth every penny spent on them." This statement expresses an opinion with which anyone who does not support funding for organ transplants would disagree.

When investigating controversial issues it is important that one be able to distinguish between statements of fact and statements of opinion. It it also important to recognize that not all statements of fact are true. They may appear to be true, but some are based on inaccurate or false information. For this activity, however, we are concerned with understanding the difference between those statements which appear to be factual and those which appear to be based primarily on opinion.

Most of the following statements are taken from the viewpoints in this chapter. Consider each statement carefully. *Mark O for any statement you believe is an opinion or interpretation of facts. Mark F for any statement you believe is a fact.*

If you are doing this activity as a member of a class or group, compare your answers with those of other class or group members. Be able to defend your answers. You may discover that others will come to different conclusions than you. Listening to the reasons others present for their answers may give you valuable insights in distinguishing between fact and opinion.

If you are reading this book alone, ask others if they agree with your answers. You too will find this interaction valuable.

O = opinion
F = fact

1. Organ transplants are an extraordinary technology.

2. Transplantable organs include the heart, liver, lung, kidney, pancreas, and cornea.

3. One year after surgery, more than 80 percent of those individuals who would have died without a donated organ are leading almost normal lives.

4. In abolishing illnesses doctors have achieved great things with human flesh, but they have not achieved anything much for the human soul.

5. One cannot actually nail down why it seems horrible that a kidney should be sold for a large sum of money, but to me these contracts have something very creepy and unpleasant about them.

6. People who are working in the field of transplantation should think very carefully about what the consequences of that sort of thing can be if it gets out of control.

7. In 1984 Congress passed a bill banning the buying or selling of organs for transplant.

8. Roughly a third of donated kidneys for transplants come from live donors.

9. In attempting to increase organ donations, the government only makes matters worse.

10. Each year, organs are taken from only 3,500 of the nation's 20,000 potential donors.

11. Society doesn't expect people to work for free; it shouldn't expect them to give organs for nothing.

12. Heart transplants are being performed at the rate of 1,200 per year.

13. Organ donations are too important to be left to the whims of altruism or the dead weight of government bureaucracy.

14. Congress should hold public hearings on the barriers that have prevented experiments involving artificial hearts.

15. The open-minded can only call the artificial heart program a failure.

16. Robert Jarvik, the inventor of the Jarvik-7, told a medical writer that he believes a stroke is an acceptable complication for the use of an artificial heart.

Periodical Bibliography

The following list of periodical articles deals with the subject matter of this chapter.

Lawrence K. Altman	"Artificial Hearts: Bold Experiments Still Have To Prove Worth," *The New York Times*, June 20, 1986.
American Medical News	"Task Force Asks Expanded Funds for Transplants," July 25, 1986.
Roger W. Evans	"Heart Transplant Dilemma," *The Washington Times*, April 29, 1986.
Tim D. Kane	"Supply, Demand, and Heart Transplants," *USA Today*, July 1986.
Bill Keller	"Gut Issues," *The New Republic*, March 19, 1984.
Betty Ann Kevles	"Transplants: The Gift of a Second Chance at Life," *Los Angeles Times*, June 18, 1986.
Dena Kleiman	"Turning Death into Life: Agonizing Decisions of Heart Transplant Unit," *The New York Times*, May 14, 1984.
John Langone	"The Artificial Heart Is Really Very Dangerous," *Discover*, June 1986.
Brendan Long	"Vital Facts About Organ Transplants," *Consumers' Research*, May 1986.
Terence Monmaney	"The Artificial Heart: Can It Save Lives?" *Science 86*, June 1986.
Mark Moran	"Acting Out Faith Through Organ Donation," *The Christian Century*, June 18/25, 1986.
Nicholas Rescher	"Whose Life Should We Save When Technology Is Scarce?" *Los Angeles Times*, March 10, 1986.
Thomas E. Starzl	"Will Live Organ Donations No Longer Be Justified?" *The Hastings Center Report*, April 1985.
Anastasia Toufexis	"Stilling the Artificial Beat," *Time*, August 18, 1986.
Amy Ward	"Putting a Price Tag on Human Organs," *Mother Jones*, December 1984.

Should Limits Be Placed on Reproductive Technology?

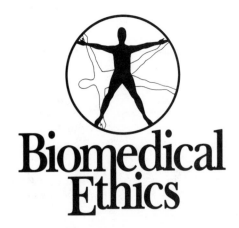

Biomedical Ethics

"*[Artificial insemination by donor] deliberately and consciously sets out to condone the restructuring of a long accepted societal norm.*"

Artificial Insemination by Donor Should Be Restricted

Charles Meyer

The Reverend R. Charles Meyer is director of the Department of Pastoral Care at St. David's Community Hospital in Austin, Texas. He has served as a prison chaplain and pastoral counselor and is the author of numerous magazine articles. In the following viewpoint, Reverend Meyer examines several ethical issues related to artificial insemination by donor (AID). He concludes that AID and other reproductive technologies should be restricted before the technologies themselves, rather than human conscience, set science's ethical boundaries.

As you read, consider the following questions:

1. According to the author, what has been the traditional objection against AID?
2. How is it now possible for a child to have five parents?
3. How does Meyer define the traditional family structure? Why does he think artificial insemination by donor families are not as good as traditional families?

Charles Meyer, "The Reproductive Revolution: Ethics of Assisted Begetting," *The Witness*, April 1986. Reprinted by permission.

With all the begetting going on in the Bible you would think there would be more commentary on the use of donor sperm. Actually much is there, mainly focusing on the *method* of that procedure. But that was in the olden days when you had to have sex to produce babies.

Biomedical assisted reproduction techniques are now offering options that will determine the kinds of families we will *construct* and the kinds of children we will choose to have (or abort). While the legal and medical ramifications of the these options are currently being debated around the country, the religious community has been reticent to study, evaluate and advise upon the ethical dilemmas inherent in them. One such area of discussion is AID—Artificial Insemination by Donor.

Children Without Sex

George Annas of The Hastings Center has noted that the technology of the '70s brought us sex without children and the technology of the '80s brings us children without sex. In addition, the '80s now offer women the option of children conceived from another man's sperm without committing what has been traditionally considered adultery.

Artificial Insemination by Donor (AID) is now a relatively common method of circumventing male infertility. When the male of a couple is found to be oligospermic (he produces too few sperm), azoospermic (no sperm) or infertile for unknown reasons, the couple can choose to have the woman receive semen from a donor. When the woman's ovulatory cycle is ready, semen collected from a donor is placed into the woman through a tube, often with the husband present.

Until recently, those who have objected to the practice of AID have done so largely on the basis of adultery, the breaking of the fidelity bond of the marriage contract. Introduction of a third party into the intimacy of the marriage was considered to be intrusive and divisive, and to separate love making from baby making, an unnatural and unwarranted act.

Others argue that, since no sexual intercourse takes place, no adultery has occurred and no bonds have been broken. In fact, they contend that the marriage bond has been strengthened both by the decision to have the procedure and by the hoped-for result of desired offspring.

But "new occasions teach new duties" and the technology of In Vitro Fertilization and Embryo Transfer (IVF-ET) is offering expanded possibilities when combined with AID. To traditional

96

critics, adultery is now the least of their worries. With AID and IVF-ET it is now possible for a child to have five parents: a genetic mother and father, a gestational mother, and a sociological mother and father (the ones who raise the child).

The following ethical dilemmas develop partly from the use of AID itself and partly from its use in combination with IVF. These issues bear careful scrutiny and cautious evaluation due to their far reaching (and as yet untested) individual and societal implications.

Donor Selection

Who ought to be chosen or accepted as appropriate semen donors? Many programs use medical students exclusively, claiming that they have "a better understanding of the process" than others. But is such an understanding required? Other programs without a pool of medical students often use law students. (Physicians are then in the rather ironic position of reproducing attorneys).

Dehumanizing Parenthood

Human parenthood is . . . . a basic form of humanity. To violate this is already dehumanizing, even if spiritualistic or personalistic or mentalistic categories are invoked to justify it . . . . The parameters of human life, which science and medicine should serve and not violate, are grounded in the . . . flesh and in the nature of human parenthood.

Paul Ramsey, quoted in *Human Medicine*, 1984.

But restricting the groups which are "acceptable" as donors seems open to the charge of elitism at best and classism at worst. What makes the semen of a medical student (or law or seminary student) any more valuable or desirable than that of a poor person who also sells blood plasma?

As a rule, U.S. donors receive $50 per donation. Ought there to be any payment at all? Does not, in fact, the word "donation" imply a free gift? How many persons would offer to go through the inconvenience of screening, selection and scheduling necessary to donate their semen without any prospect of monetary gain? . . .

Screening for Disease

Screening for disease is another important factor. Some AID programs rely solely upon the statement of the donor for information regarding health and genetic history. In July of 1985, four Australian women reportedly contracted acquired immune deficiency syndrome (AIDS) through semen donors in an artificial insemination program. Many programs, therefore, and their government overseers, are beginning to require screening for genetic diseases as well as for hepatitis and the HTLV III virus responsible for AIDS.

The role of the donor is another ethical variable. Should the receiving couple be able to choose a particular person for this service? If a husband dies can a wife choose his twin brother to donate semen in order to produce a child with nearly identical genetic characteristics? Or should the donor always be anonymous? Some programs include a waiver of rights statement signed by the donor to avoid legal problems with visitation or paternity issues. In the 22 states that have legislation covering AID, the need for a waiver is usually precluded by laws that determine the father to be the husband of the woman who bears the child, thus also circumventing the necessity for legal adoption.

But other programs invite the full participation of the semen donor into the lives of the couple and offspring. His collaboration is public and made known throughout the process, from the artificial insemination, through the hoped-for pregnancy and birth, and often into the life of the child. Sometimes the donor is responsible for regular visitation and economic support of the child. Should this be made a requirement of donors in general?

Finally, unless a program limits the number of times a donor can provide semen, offspring produced by that donor may face the problem of unknown consanguinity. One donor in Washington D.C., who had provided a large number of semen samples for various programs there, advised his children not to marry anyone from the D.C. area for just that reason. Some legislators have suggested a national registry for the keeping of donor screening information so that consanguinity can be avoided to a great degree.

Records and Research

What kinds of records should be kept? Unlike the parallel situation of adoption, AID records tend to be sparse, with little uniformity. This may be responsible, in part, for the fact that so few follow-up studies of donors, families or children exist.

Some have argued that no records should be kept at all, thus assuring the anonymity of the donor and extinguishing the possibility of family disruption caused from discovery by the child of the donor/parent. Others believe that files (including a photograph), should be carefully kept, so that if the child does want to know who the biological/genetic father was, the information is available. Such data would also make follow-up studies possible.

Research that has been done, much in the last five years, reports mixed results. Some studies show positive benefits and little harm to the AID child and couple, while others indicate potential problems with paternity questions, as well as a nearly unanimous abhorrence to telling the child "the secret" of his or her origin. Apparently no long-term developmental studies have been done on the children of AID and, because the procedure is so new, none have been carried out on the use of AID with IVF-ET participants. . . .

Couple Selection

Who ought to have access to the use of AID or AID with IVF? Everyone who desires it? Only those who can afford it? Those for whom all else has failed? Most medically accepted criteria indicate the use of AID for the treatment of male infertility: oligospermia, azoospermia, physiological impotence, sterility, or infertility of unknown origin. AID may also be considered when the male has a known inheritable genetic disease or disorder. In these cases, donor semen is used at the couple's request and/or the physician's

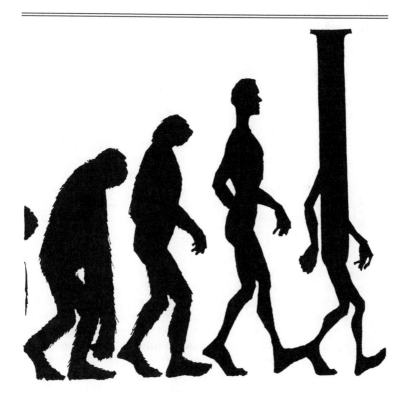

recommendation.

Similar criteria are used in selecting participants for the IVF-ET programs, though these mainly focus on female infertility. Few psychological guidelines for selection appear to be considered other than medical "necessity" and the willingness of the couple to accept either procedure. . . .

Family Structure

It is clear that the traditional family structure consists of two parents with children of their own gametes. Where that structure is changed by accident, death, disability or divorce, then other socially acceptable arrangements follow. Resulting family configurations include many variations on a theme of mixed or non-existent genetic relationships. Social vocabulary describes these mixtures as "half-brother," "stepsister," "stepfather," "adopted daughter," "ex-husband," "children by my first (second, third) wife."

In nearly all of these relationships there is some genetic investment (biological relationship) resulting from the broken bonds of the original family relationship. Supporters of AID and AID with IVF argue that using these procedures produces offspring with at least half the genes of the couple, thus bonding them closer than adoption might.

Critics counter that producing a child with half the genes of the parents results in an asymmetrical relationship. Only one member of the couple (the wife) is genetically invested and thus bonded to the offspring. In times of distress the husband may not feel responsible for "her child," or be told "It's not your child, anyway." With adoption, on the other hand, there exists a genetically symmetrical relationship. Neither parent has a genetic claim, and thus both are equally free to relate without the pressure of that claim.

The Traditional Family Model

The model for the traditional family is clear, though variations caused by unforeseen events are, of course, acceptable. Ought we, however, to deliberately restructure families away from that model by the planned introduction of a third genetic party into the couple's relationship? Does the intense desire for children with the genes of at least one parent offset the psychological and sociological implications inherent in the introduction of another's semen into the couple's family structure? Is it not the case that the desired family structure is that of two parents with children who are wanted and loved, regardless of genetic relationships? With this model as the goal, adoption and biological birthing are *equally* valuable and the pejorative nature of "infertility" itself is entirely circumvented.

As for the argument that the technologies are "unnatural," many people consider that *all* medicine is "unnatural" and thus immune from criticism on those grounds. But there does seem an immense difference between the replacement of a hip or knee joint with an artificial appliance, or the treatment of an epidemic with serum injections, and the use of AID with or without IVF. The social ramifications of most medical practices go no further than the effect upon the individual, or the individual and the family. The use of AID, especially with IVF, deliberately and consciously sets out to condone the restructuring of a long accepted societal norm.

As mentioned earlier, few long-term studies of AID and its effects on family life have been conducted and none on the use of AID with IVF. But even if sufficient data existed, ought we to participate in such technological restructuring, merely because it is possible? And does not that restructuring reinforce genetic replication as a higher value than the nurturing of children in general, thus judging infertile couples (and those who adopt) as "inferior?"

The Issue of Infertility

The medical community prefers to present AID/IVF only as the "treatment of infertility." Because they view AID as an "acceptable" standard for treatment, and IVF as becoming an acceptable standard for treatment, they largely see no reason for caution in combining the two. The technology is there, therefore it ought to be used.

But to see AID/IVF merely as an issue of infertility is evidence of professional myopia and cultural arrogance. It is, of course, true that some couples grappling with infertility feel damaged, cheated and unfulfilled. Such feelings are reinforced by a medical system that describes infertility as an illness to be treated and an abnormality to be overcome. Insurance companies also participate in this, paying for obstetrical bills (some even for several IVF attempts) but not adoption fees. Similarly, state and federal tax systems allow deductions for these medical bills but not for expenses incurred in adoption. Is such a heavy weighting in favor of novel medical approaches to infertility, and against adoption, just? . . .

No *Right* To Have Children

Some have argued that it is unjust to the infertile male not to have access to AID, and unjust to the infertile couple not to provide AID with IVF. But while there is a desperate need to have children (often based on the erroneous learned belief that infertility is a sign of personal failure) there is no *right* to have them. One has the right to attempt to have them, but children—or resources to produce them—are not owed to anyone. As J.R. Nelson stated in *The Christian Century* as early as 1982: "Calls for federal funding of IVF based on rights are as persuasive as demands for printing presses to fulfill the right of free speech."

Others believe that the uncreated embryos are done an injustice by not permitting conception and birth into the world. It is better to be born they argue, than never to have existed. But since we have no direct experience with nonexistence, the question cannot logically be answered.

Finally, even if true, the argument that life is preferable to death or nonexistence is further evidence that we ought to take seriously our first duty to those who are alive already—and available for adoption. . . .

Stating Our Preferences

One thing is clear. If we do not soon state our preferences regarding limits and boundaries appropriate for reproductive technology, the ethically unlimited and morally boundless technology will set them for us.

"[Artificial insemination by donor] may be the best solution to overcome the infertile couple's inability to have their own . . . child."

Artificial Insemination by Donor Should Be Allowed

The Ethics Committee of the American Fertility Society

The American Fertility Society is a professional medical association based in Birmingham, Alabama. The following viewpoint is taken from its Ethics Committee's statement on new reproductive technologies. In this statement, the Committee supports the use of artificial insemination by donor (AID). Despite public reservations about the introduction of a third party into the marital relationship, the Committee finds no compelling medical or ethical reasons to prohibit the use of AID.

As you read, consider the following questions:

1. According to the statement, what are some reasons for the use of donor sperm? What are some reservations about its use?
2. Why does the Committee recommend AID as a better alternative than adoption?

The Ethics Committee of the American Fertility Society, "Ethical Considerations of the New Reproductive Technologies." From *Fertility and Sterility* Vol. 46, Supplement 1, pg 36S, 1986. Reproduced with the permission of the publisher, The American Fertility Society, Birmingham, Alabama.

The use of donor semen to treat the infertile couple can be traced to the 19th century, but it was not until the late 1960s that its use expanded globally. In part, this delay was due to public opinion and to uncertainty as to whether the donor or consenting husband was the legal father. With greater public understanding of the procedure, the sharp decrease in numbers of children available for adoption, and the recognition that treatment of the infertile man is very difficult, public acceptance of artificial insemination—donor (AID) has increased.

The legal climate has also improved. For example, laws governing the paternity of the child conceived through AID have been established in 28 states, providing that the AID offspring is the legal child of the sperm recipient and her consenting husband. In states without such statutes, it is highly likely that the courts would reach the same result. It is essential, however, to obtain the consent of the husband, preferably in writing, to ensure that he will be deemed the legal father of the child.

In no case has an anonymous sperm donor been held to parental responsibility for the child created with his sperm. This is true whether or not the sperm recipient is married. "The anonymous donor of the sperm cannot be considered the 'natural father,' as he is no more responsible for the use made of his sperm than is the donor of blood or a kidney," wrote the California Supreme Court.

Reasons for Using AID

The primary reason for the use of donor sperm is to treat the infertile couple when abnormal semen findings exist in the husband and the wife is potentially fertile. Causes for male infertility include the following: (a) the husband is permanently sterile because of irreversible azoospermia, regardless of the cause; (b) the husband is sterile secondary to a vasectomy and does not wish surgical correction, or surgical correction was unsuccessful; and (c) the husband has other semen abnormalities that have failed to improve with appropriate medical treatment.

There are additional situations in which AID may be used: (a) the husband has a known hereditary or genetic disorder, such as Tay-Sachs, Huntington's disease, hemophilia, or chromosomal anomalies; (b) the husband has noncorrectable ejaculatory dysfunction secondary to illness, trauma, surgery, or medication; or (c) there has been a potentially mutagenic alteration in the husband's sperm because of exposure to ionizing radiation, chemotherapy, or other noxious agents.

Finally, the single woman may be a candidate after appropriate evaluation and counseling.

The main reservation concerning the use of AID is the uncertainty that arises with the introduction of third-party gametes into the marital unit. First, there is concern about the possibility that the procedure might create psychologic problems in the husband, wife, and/or donor, whether the donor is identified or not. Second, there is the risk of transmitting serious genetic disorders or infectious diseases by the use of donor semen. The husband is also included in this concern, because the physician may not be aware of the husband's role if an infectious disease develops in the recipient wife after AID. Some genetic disorders that should be considered and avoided include hereditary hypercholesterolemia, hemoglobin disorders, congenital hip dislocation, and multiple polyposis of the colon. The major infectious diseases to consider include Acquired Immune Deficiency Syndrome; hepatitis B, non-A and non-B hepatitis; cytomegalovirus-induced syndrome in the neonate; chlamydial salpingitis, and papilloma virus-induced disorders. In addition, there is concern about consanguinity through excessive use of the same donor.

A separate issue, mainly a psychologic one, is the effect of AID

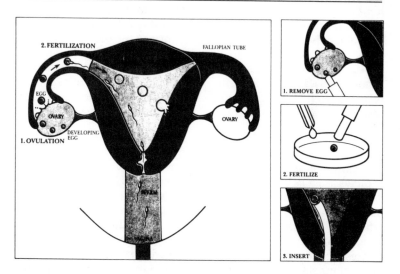

During *in vitro fertilization*, developing eggs are first surgically removed from an ovary. Second, each egg is joined with concentrated sperm sample in a culture dish, then placed in an incubator. Third, fertilized eggs are inserted through the cervix into the uterus.

Gerda Didion. Reprinted with permission.

on the resultant child, as well as on the family relationship. This includes the possibility that adverse interpersonal relationships may develop in the long term because of the perceived need to maintain secrecy concerning the child's origin. Alternatively, there is a concern that psychologic damage may result if the child learns inadvertently that AID was responsible for his or her origin. The Committee notes that there is a lack of information about whether secrecy is better for the child. . . .

The Best Solution

AID may be the best solution to overcome the infertile couple's inability to have their own combined lineal child. At least AID provides a child with a genetic link to the wife and enables the rearing parents to experience pregnancy. In addition, the available literature, although scarce, does not indicate any increase in psychologic risks due to AID.

The alternative option of adoption to bring a child into a marriage is beset with the problems of decreased numbers of available children and long waiting periods. In addition, the process of adoption has attendant legal and medical uncertainties. For example, the present concerns of society with regard to the child's right to know the details of his or her origin place a burden on both the prospective adopting parents and the mother who gives up her child for adoption. Even the biologic father may contest the adoption at some later date if his permission was not obtained. There may be a deficient medical history of the biologic parents, with resultant medical uncertainties. Also, the possibility of substance abuse may have had an adverse effect on the infant that is not readily apparent at birth. When AID is used, the risks should be minimized by the following of appropriate genetic and health screening procedures on the donor, the female recipient, and her husband.

Ethically Acceptable

Because of the general concern over the use of third-party gametes, the use of AID remains controversial. However, the Committee finds the use of AID ethically acceptable. There may be potential recipients or groups in the position to offer this service who find that the reservations to the procedure outweigh the benefits to the couple, i.e., that the procedure is not in the best interests of the persons integrally and adequately considered. In that circumstance, the recipient or group would not wish to participate in an AID program.

The Committee recommends that more emphasis be placed on the potential psychologic impact of AID. Counseling both before and after successful AID should be encouraged, rather than merely offered.

The Committee recommends that physicians furnish the couple with an adequate consent form. This form should include information on the risk, although very slight, of infectious diseases with the use of fresh semen. Although the use of frozen semen is considered to be less efficient for achieving high pregnancy rates per cycle, it is thought by many to be safer because it reduces the risks of transmitting infectious diseases.

A Permanent Record

The Committee recommends that physicians should maintain a permanent record designed to preserve anonymity and confidentiality; this record should include both identifiable and nonidentifiable health and genetic screening information. The Committee recognizes that, in most instances, these records may be released with nonidentifying information. However, in extreme situations, the release of identifying material may be required.

No Ethical Objections

AID has been widely used for many years and is not under any threat of being stopped. In the United States it has been estimated that 100,000 AID children had been born by the year 1957, and the total must now be several times that figure, with approximately 20,000 American women receiving AID each year and an estimated 10,000 to 20,000 children born via AID annually. In other Western nations, AID does not have such a long history of widespread use, but its use has increased dramatically in the past decade. . . .

We have found that AID can give rise to some ethical problems, but that on the whole it is an ethically acceptable procedure.

Peter Singer and Deane Wells, *Making Babies*, 1984.

The Committee recommends that the same donor should not be used for more than ten offspring. With this provision, the risk of consanguinity is essentially nonexistent unless population subsets are involved. Moreover, to avoid problems of inappropriate motivation on the donor's part, the Committee thinks that no payment should be made for the semen donation, although compensation for time and expenses incurred by the donor is acceptable.

Finally, the Committee recommends that scrupulous attention should be paid to the genetic and health screening of sperm donors. . . . In addition, as in other areas of obstetric practice, such screening should be offered to the recipient wife and her husband.

"Surrogacy should be a legitimate practice."

Surrogate Motherhood Should Be Permitted

Alan A. Rassaby

Surrogate motherhood, or surrogacy, is the practice of bearing another woman's child. The surrogate mother is the woman who carries the child but, upon its birth, gives it to the couple who hired her. In the following viewpoint, Alan A. Rassaby examines some of the dilemmas surrounding surrogate motherhood. Though some object to the practice on moral and social grounds, he concludes that it is legitimate. Rassaby is a Research Fellow at the Centre for Human Bioethics at Monash University in Clayton, Australia.

As you read, consider the following questions:

1. How does Rassaby define "surrogate"?
2. What, according to Rassaby, are some objections to surrogate motherhood?
3. Why does Rassaby favor surrogate motherhood?

Alan A. Rassaby, "Surrogate Motherhood: The Position and Problems of Substitutes."
© William A.W. Walters and Peter Singer 1982. Reprinted from *Test-Tube Babies* edited by William A.W. Walters and Peter Singer (1982), Oxford University Press.

And still Abram's wife Sarai bore him no children. But she had
an Egyptian maid-servant, called Agar; and now she said to her
husband, The Lord, as thou seest, denies me motherhood; Betake
thyself to this maid of mine, in the hope that I may at least have
children through her means.

Genesis 16

For most of us, the term 'surrogate motherhood' is so closely
associated with the 'new technology' that the idea that it has been
going on for many thousands of years could come as something
of a shock. It could also prove professionally embarrassing to an
army of journalists who have so recently and loudly trumpeted
the advent of a fresh challenge to our old values. One can sympathize with the jounalist who regards the tale of Abram, Sarai,
and Agar with a measure of suspicion, after all, it is not exactly
current news. At the same time, it takes us closer to the heart of
the matter.

A Substitute Mother

For the word 'surrogate' means no more than 'substitute'. A surrogate mother is a substitute mother: she is a person who, for
financial or compassionate reasons, agrees to bear a child for
someone else. A couple could conceivably enlist the services of a
surrogate mother because the female partner is unable or unwilling either to become pregnant or to carry a pregnancy to term.
A woman who suffers from a heart disease or partial paralysis
or who has a history of miscarriages could fall within this category.

For many of these couples, adoption is no longer a viable alternative because of the age of one or both of the applicants or
because of the diminishing numbers of healthy, non-handicapped
babies who are available for adoption.

Surrogate motherhood has until now taken one of two forms.
In its first form, the husband of a woman may impregnate a second woman by means of sexual intercourse (as in the story of
Abram). On birth of the child, the surrogate relinquishes custody
of the child to the couple and according to the terms of an earlier
agreement or contract under which she may receive certain financial benefits.

In its second and more publicized form, the impregnation occurs through a process of artificial insemination. This method
avoids the 'adultery aspect' present in the first variant while still
satisfying the desires of a certain number of couples to have a child
who is at least partially biologically their own. . . .

An analysis of the surrogacy debate reveals the existence of four schools of thought. In the first school are those who believe that surrogacy should be proscribed because it constitutes an unacceptable practice. In the second are those who argue that a person who has given birth to a child should not be legally forced to relinquish custody of that child to another person with whom she has contracted. A proponent of this view may or may not believe that surrogacy should be encouraged because of its positive aspect. Finally, there are those people who believe that surrogacy is inevitable and that society must protect itself and its members by regulating the process. Supporters of this alternative see no point in debating the merits or otherwise of surrogacy. Their attitude is best expressed in the words 'it's here to stay, so let's do our best with what we've got'.

Help from Medical Science

It cannot be wrong in principle to use technical means to bypass a biological or physiological barrier to parenthood. Enabling people to become biological parents is one way that nature is modified and, at the same time, fulfilled. By modifying the "natural" function of a woman's body, the natural longings for childbirth may be realized and nature's way of perpetuating the human race can be facilitated. As long as it is natural to have and want children, it cannot be unnatural or unacceptably artificial to facilitate the process by medical science.

Paul D. Simmons, *Birth and Death: Bioethical Decision-Making*, 1983.

Subscribers to the first view raise a number of objections to surrogacy. Some would argue that it encourages immorality. Dickens observes that 'a female who, especially but not only for payment, offers the services of her body for the gratification of others is so quickly vilified and named as a whore that consideration of reputable and modern analogues for the practice of embryo transfer must consciously be sought'.

To adopt this view would be to ignore the wealth of existing analogues. The wet nurse who provides milk for the suckling infant and the person who donates a kidney or other organ for use in a transplant operation are but two such samples. Nor are biblical analogues inappropriate. Just as Sarai sought to satisfy her desire for maternity through her maid-servant, Agar, so too did the barren Rachel give her maid-servant, Bala, to the Patriarch Jacob in order that 'through her means, I shall have a family of my own' (Genesis 30). Certainly in the biblical context, a woman who volunteered to have a child for another woman, far from being vilified, was blessed.

Others argue that to sanction surrogacy would be to encourage exploitation of both the surrogate and the person who seeks her services. The latter could be charged vast and unconscionable sums for these services. This would hardly seem to be a good reason to proscribe surrogacy but instead reminds us of the need for government regulation of the transaction. More commonly, ethicists object to surrogacy on the ground that the surrogate herself could be coerced into that role through poverty or unemployment. From one perspective, the surrogate can conceivably be regarded as the victim of an unfair social order. Without denying this, it seems rather counterproductive to deny her this option. Given a choice between poverty and exploitation, many people may prefer the latter. The dilemma recalls to mind the words of a friend who told me that she never gives money to intellectually handicapped children collecting from the occupants of stationary cars at traffic lights because they were underpaid and exploited by the charities that employed them. I wonder to where else these children could have looked for a source of income.

Another proposition sometimes asserted is that surrogacy may prove to be against the interests of both the surrogate mother who gives up the child and the child himself or herself. Little research has been done on the psychological and emotional bonds that tie a child to its 'birth-giving' mother and the trauma which could result on separation. If we continue to permit adoption, however, we can hardly ban surrogacy on this ground.

A Legitimate Practice

The primary benefit of surrogacy is that it would satisfy the desires and perceived needs of a number of women including those women who are unable to carry a child to term and who cannot adopt a baby because of advancing age or for some other reason. For those people, access to the services of a surrogate will become increasingly important as the numbers of babies available for adoption continue to decline. It is this social service factor which persuades me that surrogacy should be a legitimate practice. I do not think that the surrogate's receiving payment for the service detracts from its social value in any way. Nor am I persuaded by the argument that the children will be 'devalued' in the eyes of the community because they are 'bought and sold'. In most cases, the services of a surrogate will only be sought after all other viable alternatives have been exhausted. Far from being devalued, this child is likely to be especially loved. . . .

A central theme in the debate over regulation is whether access to the services of a surrogate should be restricted to those people who, for medical reasons, are unable to bear a child and should be denied to those women who, though physically capable of giving birth, do not do so either because they are too busy or because their careers require certain aesthetic standards which would not be met if they were pregnant. Lawyers have expressed conflicting views on this matter.

I do not believe that we are entitled to argue (as some have argued) that the need of the woman who physically cannot give birth is an actual one whereas the need of the busy female executive or model is more perceived than actual. To the latter, the need may be just as great as to the former. Unfortunately, one can expect there to be some discrimination in practice, however, at least in times of scarce resources. One cannot avoid the fact that society places a greater premium on a woman's childbearing role than it does on her employment prospects. A woman who physically cannot give birth will therefore be regarded with more sympathy and will be perceived to have a greater need than the woman whose vocational ambitions preclude a natural childbirth.

An Idea Whose Time Is Coming

Surrogate parenting is an idea whose time is coming. . . . I think it will replace adoption.

Noel Keane, quoted in *Making Babies*, 1984.

Another question to which consideration should be given is that of payment for the services of the surrogate. Should the parties be able to negotiate a price on a free enterprise basis or should the law regulate this aspect of the transaction by setting a recommended and a maximum fee for services? The potential for exploitation of both parties persuades me that the latter is the preferable option.

Clarifying Responsibilities

Of great importance is the need for the responsibilities of both parties to be clearly set out at the time at which the agreement is signed. Law makers must consider whether or not the surrogate mother should be responsible for any medical costs incurred during her pregnancy or whether this should be the responsibility of the genetic mother of the child. Complications during pregnancy may result in serious illness requiring a lengthy period of hospitalization. In such cases, the cost of health care or subsequent loss of income or both may be substantial. Consideration should be given, therefore, to the inclusion of a compulsory insurance scheme in the terms of every agreement. The genetic mother (or the surrogate) may be obliged to pay the premiums on the scheme.

The identity of the surrogate is also a matter of importance. Should the surrogate be required to pass a medical fitness test before and during pregnancy? Should she be required to undergo psychological assessment? Should the surrogate be forced to retire at a certain age?

One matter which clearly demands regulation is the activities of the surrogate mother during pregnancy. Should she be prohibited from smoking or drinking alcohol? What about activities which are potentially (though not intrinsically) harmful, for example, skiing? At what point does regulation become unfairly intrusive on the lives of the surrogates? What if the baby is born with a disability which can be directly attributed to an activity in which the surrogate mother engaged which was a breach of the agreement (or in breach of the law)? In such a case, should the child or his or her genetic parents have a right of action in negligence (or breach of statutory duty) against the surrogate mother?

Some writers have also discussed whether the surrogate could and should be compelled to submit to amniocentesis, and whether she can be constrained to undergo an abortion if the procedure indicates some birth defect or if the genetic parents have simply changed their minds and no longer wish to have a child. At present, legal compulsion without the consent of the surrogate would not be possible.

Giving Up the Child

At the epicentre of the dilemma is whether a surrogate mother should be legally compellable to relinquish custody of a child in favour of his or her genetic parent(s). It is one thing to recognize that a person may validly relinquish control of a child to another person who then assumes parental responsibilities in relation to the child. It is another proposition entirely to suggest that the person should be compelled to do so. . . .

The solution may be a compromise. Arguably, the long-term emotional trauma suffered by a surrogate mother who unwillingly relinquishes custody of her child may be so great that the law should adopt a special attitude to this type of contract by refusing to compel the surrogate to relinquish custody. If this is so, the law may still recognize the legitimate claim of the child's genetic mother by imposing a penalty on a surrogate who fails to fulfil her part of the bargain. Alternatively, a surrogate may be asked to leave a valuable deposit with a person or body agreed upon by both parties. The deposit could be forfeited in the event of a breach by the surrogate mother.

A much neglected facet of the debate is the issue of a right to privacy. At present, people who seek the services of a surrogate must usually enter into direct negotiations with the surrogate. Because the identity of all parties is known, privacy may become a source of great difficulty. A surrogate who changes her mind at some latter stage and who comes to 'claim' her child could cause incalculable emotional distress and damage to the child and to his or her present 'parents'. For this reason, I believe that all surrogacy contracts should be arranged through a surrogacy agency. The intervention of an agency would mean that the surrogate and the person seeking her services would have no direct contact with one another. Each would therefore remain ignorant of the identity of the other. It is essential, of course, that the agency keep a proper register of the transaction which includes the names of all parties involved. . . .

Three Options

Law makers must now choose between three options. First of all, they can ignore the storm which is gathering around the surrogacy debate and leave questions of legality to be determined on existing common law and statutory principles. Secondly, they can proscribe surrogacy by means of legislation. Thirdly, they can legislate to permit surrogacy either absolutely or subject to certain restrictions.

The first alternative is both short-sighted and impractical. It is impractical because the existing law is far from clear in its implications. It is short-sighted because it fails to take into account that a society with new technology and changing values deserves a fresh approach to questions of law reform and not one which is basted in the values of another time.

The second alternative ignores some of the benefits which surrogacy may bring. It is probably also unrealistic because it represents an attempt to proscribe what is arguably an inevitable event. Such a proscription could moreover force the practice 'underground' thereby increasing the potential for exploitation.

I believe that the solution lies in careful and detailed legislative regulation designed to promote the interests of all parties and of our society in general. One hopes that the process of law reform is set in train well before the problems grow to unmanageable proportions.

"Commercial surrogacy promotes the exploitation of women and infertile couples, and the dehumanization of babies."

Surrogate Motherhood Should Not Be Permitted

George J. Annas

George J. Annas is Utley Professor of Health Law at Boston University School of Medicine and Chief of the Health Law Section at Boston University School of Public Health. Annas argues in the following viewpoint that surrogate motherhood, the practice of bearing another woman's child, treats children like products to be bought and sold. According to Annas, surrogate motherhood is no better than baby-selling and should be illegal.

As you read, consider the following questions:

1. According to Annas, the *essence* of surrogate motherhood is not new. What does he say *is* new about surrogate motherhood?
2. Annas objects to surrogate motherhood because it is exploitive. Alan A. Rassaby, in the previous viewpoint, supports it because it solves a problem. With whom do you agree? Can you think of other arguments for or against surrogate motherhood?

George J. Annas, "At Law: The Baby Broker Boom," *The Hastings Center Report,* June 1986. © 1986 by George J. Annas. Reprinted by permission.

Should babies be treated as commodities? Should reproduction be commercialized? Should motherhood be determined by contract? A few years ago these questions seemed absurd. But the hope that surrogate motherhood would wither of its own weirdness is now beginning to seem quaint. Indeed, two recent court decisions strongly support commercial surrogate mother agreements. If surrogate mother companies were listed on the New York Stock Exchange, these cases would have sent their stock soaring.

Surrogate Parenting Associates

Almost since its inception, Surrogate Parenting Associates, Inc. (SPA) was in trouble in its home state of Kentucky. In 1981, the Attorney General instituted proceedings against the corporation to revoke its charter. He charged that by entering into commercial surrogate arrangements in which a woman would be paid to be artificially inseminated, and then to bear a child for whom she would relinquish parental rights (for later step-parent adoption by the father-sperm-donor's infertile wife), the corporation violated the state's prohibition against the "purchase of any child for the purpose of adoption." The statute was amended in 1984 to add the words, "or any other purpose, including termination of parental rights."

A trial court ruled against the Attorney General, an Appeals Court in his favor, and the Supreme Court of Kentucky has now sided with the corporation (*Surrogate Parenting Associates v. Kentucky,* 704 S.W.2d 209 [1986]). The court declared that the intention of the legislature in prohibiting baby selling was solely "to keep baby brokers from overwhelming an expectant mother or the parents of a child with financial inducements to part with the child." It therefore approved of baby sales if the price was agreed to *before* conception, and the surrogate mother retained the right to cancel the contract up to the point of relinquishing her parental rights.

Surrogate motherhood is a non-technical application of artificial insemination that requires no sophisticated medical or scientific knowledge or medical intervention. But the court saw surrogate motherhood as modern science, and did not want to interfere with "a new era of genetics," "solutions offered by science," and "new medical services."

The majority's opinion thus misses the focus of the Attorney General's argument: surrogacy's essence is not science, but commerce. The only "new" development in surrogacy is the introduction of physicians and lawyers as baby brokers who, for a fee, locate women willing to bear children by AID and hand them over to the payor-sperm donor after birth. The novelty lies in treating children like commodities.

This Justice Vance, one of two dissenting justices, understood. He noted that the corporation's "primary purpose is to locate women who will readily, for a price, allow themselves to be used as human incubators and who are willing to sell, for a price, all of their parental rights in a child thus born." His rationale was that payment is made to the surrogate in two parts. The first part "of the fee is paid in advance for the use for her body as an incubator." But the second portion of the fee is not paid unless and until "her living child is delivered to the purchaser, along with the equivalent of a bill of sale, or quitclaim deed, to wit—the judgment terminating her parental rights." As the judge persuasively argues, the last payment must be for the child, since if the child is not delivered, the last payment need not be made.

An Immoral Practice

Artificial insemination in marriage, with the use of an active element from a third person, is . . . immoral and as such is to be rejected summarily. Only marriage partners have mutual rights over their bodies for the procreation of new life, and these rights are exclusive, nontransferable and inalienable.

Pope Pius XII, quoted in *America*, December 7, 1985.

The majority probably thought it was approving very *limited* baby selling: permitting a father-sperm donor to purchase the gestational mother's interest in his genetic child if the gestational mother contracted to make such a sale prior to conception and still desires to sell her child after its birth.

Limiting Baby Buying

But limiting baby buying to fathers does not make baby buying any more tolerable than permitting a father to kidnap his biological child from its mother would make kidnapping tolerable. If mothers are to give up their parental rights to fathers, it should be *voluntarily*, and without a monetary price that converts the child into a commodity. That is what the Kentucky legislature undoubtedly had in mind when it outlawed baby selling.

The Kentucky court did not address baby selling in the case of full surrogacy: a surrogate who "gestates" an embryo to which she has made no genetic contribution. But a lower Michigan court has. Twenty-three-year-old Shannon Boff was pregnant with a child genetically unrelated to her at the time the question of her motherhood came up. .... For the first reported time in the U.S., in vitro fertilization (IVF) had been used to fertilize an ovum from an infertile woman (who lacked a uterus), and the resulting embryo was implanted into another woman, who agreed to act as a surrogate mother by gestating the fetus.

This raised an undecided legal question: Should the genetic or the gestational mother be considered the "legal" mother? That is, which woman should have legal rearing rights and responsibilities? The genetic parents, who had paid $40,000 for this "project" ($10,000 of which went to Ms. Boff) wanted to have their own names listed on the child's birth certificate, not the names of Ms. Boff and her husband.

A Set-Up Case

Unfortunately, the case was a set-up. Even though both "competing" sets of parents were represented by legal counsel, they all wanted the judge to rule the same way. Since she did, there will be no appeal and no further judicial analysis of the question. Nor did the judge appoint anyone to represent the interests of the potential child. Like the Kentucky court, the Michigan judge decided to let contracts and commerce rule the day, rather than deal with any wider social issues, or consider the best interests of any child.

In so doing, the judge consistently put form over substance. For example, in determining that Ms. Boff's husband should not be presumed to be the father of his wife's child, the judge accepted the argument of their attorney that he could not be presumed the father under the AID statute because he signed a "nonconsent to any type of artificial insemination of his wife." But given his active participation in the entire project (he said he rubbed and drew faces on his wife's enlarged stomach and treated the pregnancy as if his wife was carrying their own child), his signature is hardly the "clear and convincing evidence" the statute requires. Moreover, the entire Paternity Act under which the case was brought covers only children "born out of wedlock," so the court may have had no jurisdiction at all over this case.

The discussion of maternity is taken even less seriously. Like the Kentucky court, the Detroit judge saw her primary task as trying to make the law conform with and comfort modern science. Promoting private contract and personal profit were also seen as appropriate judicial strategies. To get to this point, the judge found it necessary to rule that the state's paternity statute must be applicable to women as well as men, to afford women "equal protection of laws."

This is, of course, true only if there are no significant differences between maternity and paternity. But if there are no significant differences, then the female gamete donor should logically be treated "equally" to a male gamete donor: the child would then

118

have *two* genetic "fathers," but would have a [gestational] mother as well. Not to so recognize the gestational mother's status dehumanizes her (and all mothers?), turning her into mere breeder stock. Of course, had Ms. Boff asserted her rights and identity as the child's mother, the judge would almost certainly have upheld her claim.

"Mama"

Slowly, one step at a time, we have been separating reproduction from sexual intercourse. Artificial insemination, in vitro fertilization, surrogate motherhood. Now, in logical sequence, we have the surrogate motherhood of an in vitro fertilization. It requires a very tiny leap, more of a hop, to imagine a future embryo created from sperm donor and egg donor, implanted into a second woman, all for adoption by a third.

Who is the mother in that case? . . .

By now, we are so far removed from nature that we need a law to determine motherhood. How odd that we find ourselves arguing about the definition of the very first word in any baby's vocabulary: "Mama."

Ellen Goodman, *Saint Paul Pioneer Press and Dispatch*, May 9, 1986.

In applying the paternity statute to maternity, the court concluded that the gestational mother (whom the court referred to as the "birthing mother"), is acting as a "human incubator for this embryo to develop." Where the incubator "contracted to do this" via IVF, and where subsequent tissue typing confirms the genetic links of the child to the gamete donors, then "the donor of the ovum, the biological mother, is to be deemed, in fact, the natural mother of this infant, as is the biological father to be deemed the natural father of this child."

The "Real" Mother

Besides putting contract above biology, this conclusion begs the question of who the child's mother is during pregnancy, and also makes identification of the child's mother at birth impossible. It thus fails to protect either the child or its mother where decisions regarding the newborn infant's care need to be made quickly. The judge dealt with this by saying that her decree would depend upon . . . tissue-typing confirming the identity of the genetic parents, a procedure that would not resolve the issue until at least a few days after the birth.

Although commerce won out in court, Ms. Boff said she would leave the baby business herself: "I'm going into retirement; any more babies coming from me are going to be keepers."

The contrary conclusion—that the woman who gestates a child should be considered the child's legal mother for all purposes—is not based on antiscience, anachronistic, or sentimental views of motherhood. Rather, it is a recognition of the gestational mother's greater biological contribution to the child, including risks and physical contributions of the nine months of pregnancy, and the need to protect the newborn by always providing it with at least one immediately identifiable parent.

The gestational mother, for example, contributes more to the child than the ovum donor does in the same way she contributes more to the child than a sperm donor does. Other considerations also argue for this traditional view of motherhood. What if there are three "competing" mothers, as happens if the genetic ovum donor is anonymous (as most sperm donors are), the gestational mother a surrogate, and the contracting rearing mother simply someone who wants to raise the child? In this scenario the only relationship the rearing mother has is monetary: she paid the surrogate a fee to gestate the embryo and give up the child. If we *really* believe money and contracts should rule, then the identity of the child's mother will depend upon contract and payment only, and both genetics and gestation (and therefore all biological ties) will be irrelevant.

The Traditional View

Since neither of these results seems reasonable, and since the traditional presumption would always provide the child with an identifiable mother who would be the same woman who biologically contributed the most, the traditional assumption should continue to be utilized, even in this "brave new world," and whether or not any contracts have been signed or any money changes hands. The Kentucky court's ruling, of course, is consistent with this view. The gestational mother could honor her prior contract, but could also change her mind and retain *her* child anytime before formally relinquishing parental rights.

Commercial surrogacy promotes the exploitation of women and infertile couples, and the dehumanization of babies. If the courts think this is a small price to pay to promote the "baby business," then it's time for state legislature to define motherhood by statute.

"Frozen embryos ought to be maintained in their frozen state for as long as they are able to survive implantation."

Destroying Human Embryos Is Immoral

David T. Ozar

Reproductive technology now allows an egg and a sperm to form an embryo outside of a woman's uterus. It also makes possible the freezing of such embryos for later use. However, not all the embryos created by scientists in laboratories are needed. What should be done with them? In the following viewpoint, David T. Ozar, Ph.D., argues that these frozen embryos should never be destroyed, whether they can be implanted in a woman's uterus or not. Dr. Ozar is associate professor of philosophy, adjunct associate professor of medicine, and director of the M.A. Program in Health Care Ethics at Loyola University of Chicago.

As you read, consider the following questions:

1. The Rios case raises many ethical questions concerning frozen embryos. What do you think should be done with the Rioses' embryos?
2. According to Ozar, what are some problems with the term "viability"?
3. What, according to Ozar, is the moral status of human embryos?

David T. Ozar, "The Case Against Thawing Unused Frozen Embryos," *The Hastings Center Report*, August 1985. Reproduced by permission. © The Hastings Center.

The Rios case made headlines [in 1984]. A millionaire couple from the United States, Mario and Elsa Rios, wanted to have children. Though each had had children by former marriages, they were unable to conceive together. In 1981 they sought the help of researchers at Queen Victoria Medical Center in Melbourne, Australia. Three of Mrs. Rios's egg cells were removed and successfully fertilized in the laboratory with sperm from an anonymous donor. One of the resulting live embryos was then implanted in Mrs. Rios's womb; the two remaining embryos were frozen to preserve them for future implantation if the first implanted embryo should abort.

The implanted embryo did spontaneously abort after about ten days but Mrs. Rios said she was not emotionally ready then to have a second embryo implanted. Some time later the Rioses went to South America to adopt a child. In the spring of 1983, Mr. and Mrs. Rios and their adopted child were killed in a crash of their private airplane (*New York Times*, October 24, 1984). . . .

Who Should Decide?

Who should decide the fate of the remaining frozen embryos? If the Rioses were still alive, it would be natural to conclude, both in law and from an ethical perspective, that they, together with the doctors and researchers involved, are the responsible parties. With the Rioses now dead, should the executors appointed for the Rioses' estate or the Rioses' heirs or possibly the state take over the Rioses' role in these decisions?

A committee convened for the purpose later recommended that the embryos be destroyed. The legislators of the state of Victoria then rejected the committee's advice and passed an amendment to another bill, calling for an attempt to have the embryos implanted in surrogate mothers and then, if they came to term, placed for adoption. There has been no further word on whether they were actually implanted. Regardless of how this aspect of the matter is resolved, the doctors and researchers, who brought the sperm and ova together and who have preserved the embryos in their frozen state, will still have a role to play. I shall assume that, for our purposes, they bear the chief ethical responsibility for unused frozen embryos.

Is the fact the Rioses are deceased of importance in determining what is the right thing to do with the remaining embryos? The answer is clearly, no. If it were determined that the embryos ought to be dealt with as pieces of property, organic goods duly owned by someone, then the fact that the Rioses are deceased means only

122

that someone else owns them. By the same token, if it were determined that the embryos ought to be treated differently from pieces of property, then they ought to be so treated regardless of who has or has not died.

A Private Decision

Suppose that the Rioses had lived, that the first implanted embryo had prospered and had been born a healthy baby, and that the Rioses had chosen to have only one child. The future of the two remaining embryos would still need to be decided. On this scenario the matter would probably have been decided privately between the Rioses and the hospital-laboratory team. A number of such decisions have undoubtedly been made in just this way, between the team and other couples. But the question is the same whether we as a community reflect on it or it is asked privately by doctors and researchers and the couples who are their patients; and its answer does not depend on the fate of Mr. and Mrs. Rios. How ought people to act, what ought people to do, in regard to unused frozen embryos?

Some might argue that this question misses the point, that the real issue concerns the morality of artificial reproductive techniques themselves, of which freezing live embryos is simply one example. From this perspective all forms of fertilization other than intercourse are profoundly unnatural and immoral. The real point would be that these embryos should not have been fertilized and frozen in the first place. We are uncertain about how to proceed rightly from this point because the parties acted immorally at the outset.

Preserve, Not Destroy

The whole point of freezing embryos is to preserve life, not destroy it. The advice of the Queen Victoria Medical Centre Ethics Committee, which includes a Roman Catholic theologian, was to freeze embryos is an attempt to preserve life. On occasions, fresh embryos cannot be transferred to the uterus because of technical difficulties or because an excess of embryos is available. Rather than destroy the embryo, we are attempting to preserve it by freezing and to transfer the embryo back to the uterus at a more favourable time. At no time . . . do we intend to destroy the embryo.

Carl Wood, W.A.W. Walters, and John F. Leeton, in *Test-Tube Babies*, 1982.

This approach raises important questions about the reproductive technology that was offered to the Rioses. But this response is of little help to those who must now determine what to do about existing frozen embryos. Even if the acts that brought us to this pass were profoundly immoral, what we do next is still not a morally indifferent matter.

In trying to answer this question, it is natural to examine the lines of thought that have been developed regarding our obligations toward fetuses. Unfortunately, many of these lines tell us little about a frozen eight- or sixteen-celled embryo. For example, any obligations that we might have toward a fetus by reason of its possession of neurological functions, and hence its possession of the beginnings of the most distinctive functions of the human species, would not apply to an embryo whose cells have not yet begun to differentiate in terms of function. Even less could an embryo pass the test of actually engaging in acts of thinking, planning, choosing, or of being conscious and experiencing emotion, which some authors have made the key to a being's having rights and the rest of us having corresponding obligations.

Viability

One approach that might seem helpful here focuses on viability outside the womb. The frozen embryo is obviously outside the womb and it is not dead or dying. Indeed it is being preserved in its frozen state precisely because of its potential for continued life.

Viability is one of the criteria employed by the United States Supreme Court in the ethical justification of the legal ruling in its landmark abortion decision. In *Roe v. Wade*, the Court held that the fetus is not a legal person, a bearer of legal rights, including the legal right not to be killed, at any point from conception until the moment of live birth. But the Court held that the state does have an "interest" in "protecting the potentiality of human life," and that this interest grows "in substantiality as the woman approaches term." Moreover, at some point in the pregnancy, the Court held, this interest may be considered "compelling," that is, sufficiently important that it may outweigh other fundamental values, in this case the mother's constitutional right to control her own body and thus to seek an abortion if she chooses.

The point at which the state's interest in protecting the potentiality of human life becomes "compelling," said the *Roe* Court, is "viability." Viability is in turn described as "the capability of meaningful life outside the womb"; but the term "meaningful" is not further defined by the *Roe* Court, so the Court's understanding of viability was still unclear. In *Danforth*, however, the Court upheld a Missouri statute containing this definition of viability: "that stage of fetal development when the life of the unborn child may be continued indefinitely outside of the womb by natural or artificial life-support systems."

But as Justice Sandra Day O'Connor has argued, there is still ambiguity here. In a dissent to the Court's 1983 *Akron* decision, Justice O'Connor argues that "neither sound constitutional theory nor our need to decide cases based on the application of neutral principles can accommodate an analytic framework that varies according to the 'stages' of pregnancy, where those stages, and their concomitant standards of review, differ according to the level of medical technology at a particular time. . . . The *Roe* framework is clearly on a collision course with itself. As the medical risks of various abortion procedures decrease, the point at which the state may regulate for reasons of maternal health is moved further forward to actual childbirth. As medical science becomes better able to provide for the separate existence of the fetus, the point of viability is moved further back toward conception. . . ." Thus if medical science had developed an artificial womb, in which embryos could develop until they could live independently, the Rioses' frozen embryos would be viable under the *Danforth* definition.

Respect Should Prevail

There is an inconsistency in re-introducing a new kind of arbitrariness in allowing excess embryos to be brought into being which cannot be implanted and which must be disposed of. . . .

There are serious reasons for according these beings respect of a personal quality. There is no clear conflict with the respect due to other persons. Therefore, that respect should prevail and shape our behaviour towards these beings.

The creation of excess embryos and their consequent, inevitable destruction is discordant with such respect.

Brian Johnstone, in *Test-Tube Babies*, 1982.

But lacking an artificial womb, what are we to say? The most likely interpretation is that "life" in these definitions means not only that the organism under consideration is not dying, but also that it is able to continue to perform life functions (with or without mechanical assistance) outside of a womb. On this interpretation, the frozen embryo is not viable. For, while capable in their frozen state of not dying, these embryos cannot continue to perform life functions, even simple cell divisions, independent of the nutritive and protective environment of a woman's womb.

Competing Rights

Consequently, to return to *Roe v. Wade*, the state would not have a "compelling" interest in protecting the potential life of frozen embryos. That is, the state's interest in protecting their potential life could not outweigh the fundamental constitutional right of a woman to control her own body. But in the case of frozen embryos, no woman is involved, and thus no woman's right to control her body. Might the state's interest then be strong enough to protect frozen embryos' lives? Here the competing rights would have to be the property rights of those who own the equipment that preserves the embryos' lives. Is the state's interest in protecting the potential life of the embryo great enough to outweigh the equipment owners' rights to control their property? Or are the frozen embryos to be considered property themselves, so that their owners may dispose of them more or less as they wish, and their lives would not have any special weight in relation to the property rights of the owners of the equipment? Obviously we are now asking questions that cannot be resolved in terms of the criterion of viability. So it turns out that this criterion, like the others mentioned above, cannot resolve our question about how to act rightly toward unused frozen embryos.

But there are two approaches to our obligations toward fetuses that are informative regarding frozen embryos as well. First is the most inclusive moral position regarding obligations toward the unborn—the position that holds that the conceptus has a moral right not to be killed, and the rest of us have a moral obligation not to kill the conceptus or to intend to kill it, from the first instant of its conception. (This right, stated more completely, is a right not to be *directly* killed, and the obligation is an obligation not to *directly* kill or to intend to *directly* kill the conceptus. The added term, "directly," is very important in other contexts; but it is not important in the present discussion, and therefore I shall use the more simplified statement.)

The Instant of Conception

This position is commonly called the "right to life" position; but I shall call it the "instant of conception" position. Many other positions on these matters affirm life-related rights, including rights not to be killed under various sets of circumstances. In calling it the "instant of conception" position, I am focusing on what is truly distinctive about it and on its substantive claims in the present discussion.

According to this position, a frozen embryo, as the fruit of human conception, has a moral right not to be killed. Therefore the doctors and researchers responsible for the care of such an embryo could not morally place it in an environment known to be lethal to it. This would preclude deliberately permitting a frozen embryo to be thawed without placing it in the only environment in which it could survive thawing, namely, a woman's womb. Nor could the parents (by any definition) or anyone else morally choose that a frozen embryo be dealt with in this way.

At the same time, the "instant of conception" position provides no basis for saying that an embryo has a moral right to be implanted in a womb. The moral right not to be killed does not automatically imply a right to the use of a womb. For an embryo may be implanted in a womb only by the free choice of the woman whose womb it is. Thus the obligation not to kill an embryo does not necessarily imply an obligation on anyone's part to offer her womb for its survival. . . .

Genetic Obligation

There are then two possibilities. If no one volunteers her womb for the implantation of the unused frozen embryo, those responsible for its care will fulfill their obligations simply by not killing it, that is, by keeping it frozen. If, on the other hand, someone does volunteer for its implantation, the responsible parties would need to determine whether implantation in the womb of this particular volunteer would give the embryo a reasonable chance of survival and further development, as compared with continued freezing and the possibility of implantation in a future volunteer with more likelihood of success. It would be appropriate, also, for the responsible parties to seek out women who might desire to volunteer for implantation of unused embryos.

Wrong To Destroy

It is wrong to create something with the potential for becoming a human person and then deliberately to destroy it.

The Warnock Report, quoted in *American Medical News*, June 6, 1986.

Since frozen embryos may deteriorate over time, let us assume that there is a point at which the hospital-laboratory team can accurately say that a particular embryo is no longer able to survive implantation. Such an embryo no longer has any potential for continued life. Because it is still frozen, it is not yet dead; yet death is its only conceivable prospect. I believe that the "instant of conception" position would conclude that such an embryo no longer has any moral right that would require its continued maintenance in the frozen state. Its condition is now analogous to that of someone who is irreversibly in the process of dying. The embryo may morally be thawed at this point, and the irreversible process of its death permitted to proceed to its conclusion.

Moral Rights of Embryos

The obligations that I have just outlined, based as they are on the most inclusive position regarding our obligations to the unborn, constitute the most extensive set of obligations toward unused frozen embryos that can reasonably be defended. Next we must ask: Is any lesser set of obligations toward unused frozen embryos more reasonable? In order to respond, I shall look at a position that accords no moral rights at all to the unborn.

If a frozen embryo has no moral rights of its own, if it is more like a piece of property (or is just like a piece of property) rather than a bearer of rights, still those who are responsible for it will have obligations regarding its use and the consequences of its use. If certain ways of dealing with it would lead to significantly more good than other ways, at relatively little cost in human effort, in monetary resources, and so on, then the responsible parties would be obligated to choose those ways of acting. If certain ways of acting would involve risk of significant harm, which could be avoided at relatively little cost in human effort, in monetary resources, and so on, then the responsible parties would be obligated to avoid them.

These straightforward moral principles point to the same conclusion as is defended by the "instant of conception" position, even if the embryo has no moral rights at all. My argument follows a pattern developed by Mary Anne Warren in a famous postscript to "On the Moral and Legal Status of Abortion." In response to criticisms that her criteria for having moral rights were so strict as to deny moral rights to infants, Warren argued that even when no moral rights are relevant, morality may require that human life be preserved and protected because of the negative consequences of doing otherwise.

Costs and Benefits

Once the original outlay of expense and effort for freezing embryos has been made, embryos can be maintained in their frozen state at very little cost, in dollars or in human effort. Therefore if there are women who desire to bear a child and who might be successfully implanted with embryos unused by others, the moral principles just articulated argue strongly for maintaining unused embryos in their frozen state until they can be implanted. The costs of doing this are very small and the benefits to the mothers concerned (as well as to their spouses and other affected parties) are very great. In fact, if the good of enabling women to bear children can justify the sizable expense of developing or purchasing this technology in the first place, then it surely can justify the far smaller expense of maintaining unused embryos until other women who desire to bear a child have volunteered. It would also be reasonable for the doctors and researchers to seek out such women, especially if the frozen embryo does deteriorate over time, in the interests of maximizing the benefits and minimizing the costs of the process.

This same conclusion—that unused frozen embryos ought to be maintained in their frozen state for as long as they are able to survive implantation—can be reached in another way, which takes account of other consequences of the process. For even if frozen embryos do not have moral rights, they are still members of the human species with a potential for a full human life. Indeed it is precisely because of that potential that they were frozen in the first place. Consequently if hospital-laboratory teams, parents, or other responsible parties routinely followed a policy of simply disposing of unused frozen embryos, such a policy, if widely known, could have a negative impact on the ways in which we as individuals and as a community value and deal with human life generally, especially in other members of our species whose lives are in some way compromised. . . .

A Better Course of Action

Only reasons of economy and efficiency support a policy of disposal. But a policy of maintaining the lives of frozen embryos for as long as they could survive implantation and of actively seeking out women who might desire to bear them would be far less expensive than the setup costs of the technology that enabled us to freeze embryos in the first place. Thus, given the possible negative impact of disposing of human embryos for reasons of efficiency and economics, clearly the far better course of action is to maintain the frozen embryos until they can no longer survive implantation and to actively support their implantation when women desiring to bear them volunteer. This course of action avoids risk of significant harm at relatively little cost.

From this it is clear that those who would accord to frozen embryos no moral rights whatsoever, but who would still be guided in their obligations by consideration of the outcomes of their actions, would reach the same conclusion regarding unused frozen embryos as those who affirm the embryos' moral rights from the instant of conception. From both perspectives, as well as each of the intermediate moral positions, the responsible parties have an obligation to preserve the frozen embryos in their frozen state until such time as they can no longer survive implantation. In addition, they should support implantation of unused embryos in women who volunteer to bear them and should make reasonable efforts to locate such women when there are implantable embryos.

"There is no moral obligation to preserve the life of the embryo."

Destroying Human Embryos Is Acceptable

Helga Kuhse and Peter Singer

Helga Kuhse is a Research Fellow at the Centre for Human Bioethics at Monash University in Clayton, Australia. Peter Singer is chairman of the Department of Philosophy at the same university. In the following viewpoint, Kuhse and Singer begin with the premise that it is not wrong to destroy a human egg or sperm. They argue that human embryos, which are merely the joining of egg and sperm, may be destroyed if they are not implanted in a womb.

As you read, consider the following questions:

1. What restrictions do Kuhse and Singer place on their definition of "embryo"?
2. List the three arguments against destroying embryos cited by the authors. How do the authors refute these arguments?
3. According to the authors, how does the anti-abortion argument relate to the moral rights of embryos?

Helga Kuhse and Peter Singer, "The Moral Status of the Embryo." © William A.W. Walters and Peter Singer 1982. Reprinted from *Test-Tube Babies* edited by William A.W. Walters and Peter Singer (1982), Oxford University Press.

A living human embryo comes into existence as soon as a human egg and sperm have joined together. If the embryo is then implanted into the mother, it cannot be objected that the embryo has been denied any respect that might be due to it, for it has been placed into the environment that gives it the greatest possible chance of survival. But what if more eggs have been fertilized than can be re-implanted? What is to be done with them? Should they be frozen? But what if the couple who provided the egg and sperm do not wish to have the excess embryos re-implanted into the woman? (Perhaps the first embryo developed successfully, and they do not want any more children.) And what if, while not wishing to use the embryo themselves, the couple also do not like the idea of their genetic material being used by another couple? Should the embryos then be kept frozen forever? What point would there be in that? Or can these excess embryos simply be tipped down the sink?

Many people find such questions bewildering. Seeing no way of answering them, they throw up their hands and say, 'It's all up to the individual's subjective judgement.' Our aim is to show that there is a rational answer to these questions, which should carry conviction with everyone who accepts one very widely held premise: that it is not wrong to destroy either the egg or the sperm before they have united.

No Obligation to Embryos

On the basis of this premise we shall argue that there is no moral obligation to preserve the life of the embryo. Our argument applies specifically to the very early kind of embryo produced by the IVF programme. In other words, we are talking about an embryo that has developed for only some hours or at the most a day or two. It will only have divided a few times, into two, four, eight, or sixteen cells. (Technically, this is known as a zygote, but we shall continue to refer to it by the more widely known term 'embryo'.) At this stage, of course, the embryo has no brain, or even a nervous system. (Even the brain of a tadpole has more than 5000 cells.) The embryo could not possibly feel anything or be conscious in any way. Therefore, what we shall argue about this kind of embryo has no *necessary* application to an embryo at a later stage of development, for example, at a stage of development at which it does have a brain, and could feel pain.

Our argument begins from the premise that is is not wrong to destroy either the egg or the sperm—the gametes, as they are collectively known—before they have united. We do not know of anyone who seriously asserts that the moral status of the egg and sperm before fertilization is such that it is wrong to destroy them. For instance, if a man is asked to produce a specimen of semen so that it can be tested to see if he is fertile, no one objects to the semen being tipped out once the test is complete. And after all, in our normal lives eggs and sperm are constantly being wasted. Every normal female between puberty and menopause wastes an egg each month that she does not become pregnant; and after puberty every normal male wastes millions of sperm in sexual intercourse in which contraceptives are used, or in which the woman is not fertile; and the same applies when he masturbates or has a nocturnal emission. Does anyone regard all of this as a terrible tragedy? Not to our knowledge; and so we do not think the premise of our argument is likely to be challenged.

The Embryo Should Be Destroyed

Embryos should only be frozen with the informed consent of both gamete donors, and only for a specific and specified purpose. When the purpose is fulfilled, the frozen embryo should be destroyed.

George J. Annas, *The Hastings Center Report*, October 1984.

We shall consider some imaginary stories. They do not describe any actual occurrences or even probable ones. We are using them to illustrate a moral point.

First Story

Doctors working on an IVF programme have obtained a fertile egg from a patient and some semen from the patient's husband. They are just about to drop the semen into the glass dish containing the egg, when the doctor in charge of the patient calls to say that he has discovered that she has a medical condition which makes pregnancy impossible. The egg could be fertilized and returned to the womb, but implantation would not occur. The embryo would die and be expelled during the women's next monthly cycle. There is therefore no point in proceeding to fertilize the egg. So the egg and semen are tipped, separately, down the sink.

In accordance with our premise, as far as the moral status of the egg or the sperm before they have united is concerned, nothing wrong has been done.

Second Story

Everything happens exactly as in the first story, except that the doctor in charge of the patient calls with the bad news just *after* the egg and sperm have been placed in the glass dish and fertilization has already taken place. The couple are asked if they are prepared to consent to the newly created embryo being frozen to be implanted into someone else, but they are adamant that they do not want their genetic material to become someone else's child. Nor is there any prospect of the woman's condition ever changing, so there is no point in freezing the embryo in the hope of re-implanting it in her at a later date. The couple ask that the embryo be disposed of as soon as possible.

If the embryo has a special moral status that makes it wrong to destroy it, it would be wrong to comply with the couple's request. What, then, *should* be done with the embryo?

How plausible is the belief that it was not wrong to dispose of the egg and sperm separately but would be wrong to dispose of them after they have united? For those who believe that there is a real distinction between the two stories, here is a third story, not to be taken too seriously, but intended to bring out the peculiarity of that belief.

Third Story

This story begins just as the first one does. The doctor's call comes before the egg and sperm have been united, and so they are tipped, separately, down the sink. But as luck would have it, the sink is blocked by a surgical dressing. As a result, the egg has not actually gone down the drainpipe before the semen is thrown on top of it. A nurse is about to clear the blockage and flush them both away when a thought occurs to her: perhaps the egg has been fertilized by the semen that was thrown on top of it! If that has happened, or if there is even a significant chance of that having happened, those who believe that the embryo has a special moral status which makes it wrong to destroy it must now believe that it would be wrong to clear the blockage; instead the egg must now be rescued from the sink, checked to see if fertilization has occurred, and if it has, efforts should presumably to made to keep it alive.

On what grounds could one try to defend the view that the coming together of the egg and sperm makes such a crucial difference to the way in which they ought to be treated? We shall consider three possible grounds which have been put forward.

The Anti-Abortion Argument

The claim that a human life exists from the moment of conception is often used as an argument against abortion. We are not here considering the issue of abortion but rather the moral status of the embryo. Nevertheless, the claim is relevant to our topic, because it is often assumed that once it is acknowledged that a human life exists from the moment of conception, it will also have to be conceded that from the moment of conception the embryo has the same basic right to life as normal human beings after birth.

To assess the claim that a human life exists from conception, it is necessary to distinguish two possible senses of the term 'human being'. One sense is strictly biological: a human being is a member of the species *homo sapiens*. The other is more restricted: a human being is a being possessing, at least at a minimal level, the capacities distinctive of our species which include consciousness, the ability to be aware of one's surroundings, to be able to relate to others, perhaps even rationality and self-consciousness.

Not a Person

The preembryo deserves respect greater than that accorded to human tissue but not the respect accorded to actual persons. The preembryo is due greater respect than other human tissue because of its potential to become a person and because of its symbolic meaning for many people. Yet, it should not be treated as a person, because it has not yet developed the features of personhood, is not yet established as developmentally individual, and may never realize its biologic potential.

The Ethics Committee of The American Fertility Society, *Ethical Considerations of the New Reproductive Technologies*, September 1986.

When opponents of abortion say that the embryo is a living human being from conception onwards, all they can possibly mean is that the embryo is a living member of the species *homo sapiens*. This is all that can be established as a scientific fact. But is this also the sense in which every 'human being' has a right to life? We think not. To claim that every 'human being' has a right to life solely because it is biologically a member of the species *homo sapiens* is to make species membership the basis of rights. This is as indefensible as making race membership the basis of rights. It is the form of prejudice one of us has elsewhere referred to as 'speciesism', a prejudice in favour of members of one's own species, simply because they are members of one's own species. The logic of this prejudice runs parallel to the logic of the racist who is prejudiced in favour of members of his race simply because they are members of his race. If we are to attribute rights on morally defensible grounds, we must base them on some morally relevant characteristic of the beings to whom we attribute rights. Examples of such morally relevant characteristics would be consciousness, autonomy, rationality, and so on, but not race or species.

Hence, although it may be possible to claim with strict literal accuracy that a human life exists from conception, it is not possible to claim that a human life exists from conception in the sense of a being which possesses, even at the most minimal level, the capacities distinctive of most human beings. Yet it is on the possession of these capacities that the attribution of a right to life, or of any other special moral status, must be based.

It may be admitted that the embryo consisting of no more than sixteen cells cannot be said to be entitled to any special moral status because of any characteristics it actually possesses. It is, once again, far inferior to a tadpole in respect of all characteristics that could be regarded as morally relevant. But what of its potential? Unlike a tadpole, it has the potential to develop into a normal human being, with a high degree of rationality, self-consciousness, autonomy, and so on. Can this potential justify the belief that the embryo is entitled to a special moral status?

We believe it cannot, for the following reason. Everything that can be said about the potential of the embryo can also be said about the potential of the egg and sperm. The egg and sperm, if united, also have the potential to develop into a normal human being, with a high degree of rationality, self-consciousness, autonomy, and so on. On the basis of our premise that the egg and sperm separately have no special moral status, it seems impossible to use the potential of the embryo as a ground for giving it special moral status.

It is, of course, true that something may go wrong. The egg may be surrounded by semen, and yet not be fertilized. But it is also true that something may go wrong with the development of the embryo. It may fail to implant. It may implant but spontaneously abort. And so on. There is a possibility of something going wrong at every stage, from the production of egg and sperm right through to the time at which there is a rational and self-conscious being. That there is one more stage that the egg and sperm must go through, compared to the embryo, can scarcely make a decisive difference.

The Uniqueness of the Embryo Argument

Some will concede that there is a sense in which both the embryo and the egg and sperm, taken separately, have the same potential, namely the potential to develop into a mature human being. Yet, they will want to say, there is a difference between these two forms of potential. As long as the egg and sperm are separate, the genetic nature of the individual human being that may come to exist is still to be determined. We have no way of telling which of the hundreds of thousands of sperm in a drop of semen will fertilize the egg. The unique genetic constitution of the embryo, on the other hand, has been determined for all time.

Can this difference provide a reason for giving the embryo higher status than the egg and sperm? Surely not, for the difference still does not show that the embryo has a different potential from the egg and sperm. The egg and sperm has the potential to develop into a mature human being. There are no genetically indeterminate human beings, and every genetically determinate human being is unique, with the exception of identical twins, triplets, and so on. Thus, the uniqueness of the embryo is nothing *additional* to its potential for becoming human. Why should our inability to tell which sperm will fertilize the egg make such a difference? If we were better able to predict which sperm would fertilize the egg, would we then say that the egg and sperm were now entitled to the same moral status as the embryo? . . .

No Special Moral Status

Since none of these three grounds suffice to support a sharp distinction between the moral status of the embryo and that of the egg and sperm, we are left with just three possibilities: we must find another plausible reason for making this distinction, or we must abandon our initial premise, which was that the egg and sperm are not entitled to a special moral status which would make it wrong to destroy them, or we must hold that the embryo in its very earliest stage of life is also not entitled to a special moral status which would make it wrong to destroy it. We can find no other plausible reason for making the distinction. Our premise still seems well grounded. Hence we conclude that the newly created embryo is not entitled to a special moral status which makes it wrong to destroy it. . . .

The view we have argued for justifies the common sense reaction which we believe most readers will have had to the three stories we told earlier. If you felt that it would be absurd to hold that the medical staff are under a moral obligation to try to rescue the egg that may have been accidentally fertilized in the blocked sink, you were right. Similarly, whether the doctor's call came a minute before the egg and sperm were to be united, or a minute afterwards, makes no crucial difference. In none of these cases has a being come into existence which is capable of feeling or experiencing anything at all. In none of these cases is there a being that has a right to life.

Distinguishing Bias from Reason

Biomedical issues often generate great emotional responses in people. When dealing with such highly controversial subjects, many will allow their feelings to dominate their powers of reason. Thus, one of the most important critical thinking skills is the ability to distinguish between statements based upon emotion and those based upon a rational consideration of the facts.

Most of the following statements are taken from the viewpoints in this chapter. Consider each statement carefully. *Mark R for any statement you believe is based on reason or a rational consideration of the facts. Mark B for any statement you believe is based on bias, prejudice, or emotion. Mark I for any statement you think is impossible to judge.*

If you are doing this exercise as a member of a class or group, compare your answers with those of other class or group members. Be able to explain your answers. You may discover that others will come to different conclusions than you. Listening to the reasons others present for their answers may give you valuable insights in distinguishing between bias and reason.

If you are reading this book alone, ask others if they agree with your answers. You will find this interaction valuable also.

R = *a statement based upon reason*
B = *a statement based upon bias*
I = *a statement impossible to judge*

137

1. It does not follow that just because a technology exists, it should be used.

2. To see artificial insemination by donor merely as an issue of infertility is evidence of professional myopia and cultural arrogance.

3. One may have the right to *attempt* to have children, but children are not necessarily owed to anyone.

4. Calls for federal funding of *in vitro* fertilization based on rights are as persuasive as demands for printing presses to fulfill the right of free speech.

5. It is better to be born, some argue, than never to have existed. But since we have no direct experience with nonexistence, the question cannot logically be answered.

6. The old way of adoption to bring a child into a marriage is much less satisfactory than the innovative technology of surrogate motherhood.

7. Surrogacy is inevitable. It's here to stay, so let's do our best with what we've got.

8. If one accepts the premise that the wet nurse who provides milk for the suckling infant is analogous to the surrogate mother, and if one does not object to the former practice, then one cannot object to the latter.

9. If society places a greater premium on a woman's childbearing role than it does on her employment prospects, then a woman who physically cannot give birth will be regarded with more sympathy than the woman whose vocational ambitions preclude a natural childbirth.

10. A female who offers the services of her body for the gratification of others is quickly vilified and named as a whore.

11. If there are no significant differences between maternity and paternity, then the female who donates an egg should be treated equally to the male who donates sperm.

12. If surrogacy was permitted in the Bible, it should certainly be acceptable now.

13. The hope that surrogate motherhood would wither of its own weirdness is now beginning to seem quaint.

Periodical Bibliography

The following list of periodical articles deals with the subject matter of this chapter.

Lori B. Andrews — "Yours, Mine and Theirs," *Psychology Today*, December 1984.

Rita Arditti — "Reproductive Engineering and the Social Control of Women," *Radical America*, November/December 1985.

Rochelle Distelheim — "Test Tube Babies," *Glamour*, May 1986.

Suzanne Fields — "Could Sex Become Extinct?" *The Washington Times*, March 13, 1986.

Eileen P. Flynn — "Fashioning the Wanted Child," *Commonweal*, March 14, 1986.

David Gelman and Daniel Shapiro — "Infertility: Babies by Contract," *Newsweek*, November 4, 1985.

Diane M. Gianelli — "Go Slow on Surrogate Motherhood," *American Medical News*, September 19, 1986.

Michael Gold — "Franchising Test-Tube Babies," *Science 86*, April 1986.

Richard Lacayo — "Is the Womb a Rentable Space?" *Time*, September 22, 1986.

Aric Press with Carl Robinson — "Troubling Test-Tube Legacy," *Newsweek*, July 2, 1984.

Philip Reilly — "Study Broadens Base of Fertilization Work," *American Medical News*, June 6, 1986.

Curtis J. Sitomer — "Will the Legal Meaning of 'Parent' Change?" *The Christian Science Monitor*, August 28, 1986.

Sara Terry — "Will New Technology Redefine the Family?" *The Christian Science Monitor*, August 28, 1986.

Colin J.H. Thomson — "Australia: In Vitro Fertilization and More," *The Hastings Center Report*, December 1984.

William J. Winslade and Judith Wilson Ross — "High-Tech Babies: A Growth Industry," *The New York Times*, February 21, 1986.

Should Animals Be Used in Scientific Research?

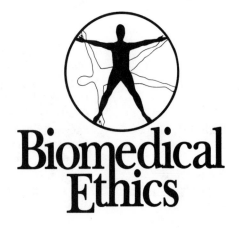

Biomedical Ethics

"Human welfare is a more vital concern than animal welfare and deserves more of our dedication because humans are more important than animals."

The Case for Animal Experimentation

Michael Allen Fox

In the last decade, animal experimentation has become more publicized and more controversial. Gruesome photos in magazines and books depict animals forcibly restrained, or with their bodies maimed, living in small, crowded cages. Some more radical commentators have suggested that animal experimentation is never justified. In the following viewpoint, Michael Allen Fox argues that these critics do not acknowledge a simple truth: human beings are more important than animals. While there must be guidelines on how animals are to be used in the laboratory, ending animal research would be devastating to human beings. He concludes that the tangible benefits of this research far outweigh the animals' discomfort. Fox is a professor of philosophy at Queen's University in Kingston, Ohio.

As you read, consider the following questions:

1. What does Fox argue is a reasonable position toward animal experimentation?
2. To what issue does the author believe antivivisectionists should devote their energy?

Michael Allen Fox, *The Case for Animal Experimentation*. Berkeley, CA: University of California Press. © 1986 The Regents of the University of California. Reprinted by permission.

This ... is an essay in support of the use of animals for human ends. Not just any animals and not just any ends, and most important of all, not without important qualifications. This is a view with which the majority of readers would probably agree. Why, then, is it necessary to ... defend it? There are two main reasons. One is that a new generation of dedicated antivivisectionists are presenting a very one-sided, often distorted picture of animal welfare issues, focusing on animal suffering in scientific research and devoting little or no attention to current intensive efforts to maintain and improve the standards of animal care or to the benefits gained from such research. Media attention everywhere is, as always, easily and frequently captured by emotional appeals on behalf of animals and by sensationalistic tactics like "guerrilla" raids on scientific laboratories aimed at "liberating" experimental animals and exposing them to the press and TV.

Soliciting an Emotional Response

This sort of behavior is unfortunately characteristic of our age, and is clearly calculated to have shock value and to polarize public opinion. There is, of course, always great danger in a populace that reacts without thinking, but the aim of many zealots promoting one cause or another is to create a widespread, intense emotional response backed by a spurious sense of moral superiority. Responsible members of the "animals rights" movement, however, have condemned these acts of violence and vandalism and have presented their ideas in a more dispassionate manner, appealing instead to argument and moral and political suasion. But in general, the public, which eventually has to make the decisions affecting, for example, the future of scientific research and to accept the consequences of such decisions (such as better or inferior standards of health care), has heard in recent times only that side of the argument that advocates the moral equality of all species and focuses on human guilt for causing animal suffering.

In the face of these influences, it is important to develop a reasonable position in support of what most human beings have believed and practiced for thousands of years—that animals are *not* our moral equals and that therefore there is no compelling ground for treating them as such. We do not have to possess the sensitivity of a St. Francis of Assisi or an Albert Schweitzer to be aware that animals are capable of suffering greatly, that some are remarkably like us in important respects, and that countless abuses of animals occur daily in every part of the world. These facts obviously have to be taken into account in arriving at a satisfactory position on our use and treatment of animals; but it does not follow, as I try to show, that a traditional, anthropocentric interpretation of morality and of humans' relationship to other species cannot be maintained. No doubt many animal welfarists and antivivisectionists will react to this position with extreme disfavor, dismissing it as essentially conservative or even reactionary. I would prefer to think of it as an antidote to extremism of all sorts—as sensible, middle-of-the-road point of view for which adequate support can be given.

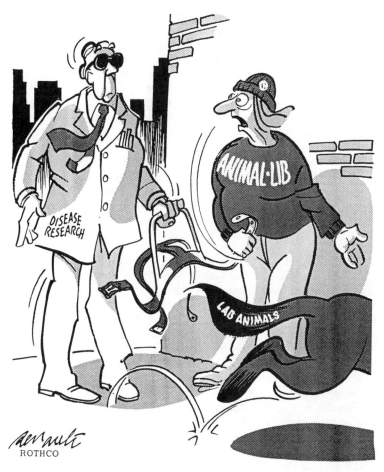

"YOU SHOULD BE ASHAMED OF YOURSELF FOR EXPLOITING THIS ANIMAL!"

Perhaps we should pause to ask what is to count as an "animal"—lions, whales, armadillos, zebras, and mice, surely; even oysters, ants, butterflies, and mosquitoes if we are willing to stretch our concept a bit. But what about viruses, bacteria, and other primitive or single-cell organisms? Where do we draw the line? It will do no good to protest that *everyone knows* what animals are and that therefore some of these examples are farfetched. In common usage anything living that is not a plant is an animal; and the universally accepted system of biological classification used by scientists includes among the animal phyla, or major divisions, everything from protozoans, sponges, and annelids (insects, scorpions, earthworms, leeches, and the like) to chordates (all organisms with vertebrae). The animal kingdom thus runs the gamut from species that respond to stimuli but are very rudimentary in function and structure, lacking a nervous system altogether (amoebas, sea cucumbers, certain molluscs) through those that are sentient and possess some limited mode of consciousness (fish, insects, reptiles, birds) to those with large and highly complex brains, highly evolved nervous systems, a wide range of social and communicative behaviors, sophisticated problem-solving capacities, and so on (chimpanzees, dolphins, humans). Exactly which of these characteristics make a species an object of our moral concern is a moot point; but even if all living things are in a sense such objects, the degree of concern that is appropriate to each species is surely a function of how we regard the characteristics it possesses. . . .

"Pathetic Fallacy"

A great deal of what has been said and written about the moral status of animals over the past two decades is characterized by sentimentalism and exemplifies the "pathetic fallacy," or the illegitimate attribution of human qualities to nature. Sentimentalism appears in two guises: the plain, old-fashioned, tug-at-the-heartstrings type and the modern, intellectualized variety. The latter is frequently present in the work of the speculative ecologists, theologians, and academics who have joined the animal rights movement but appear to possess scanty firsthand knowledge of animals or the uses to which they are put by humans. These tendencies are so commonplace now that they form part of a shared ambience, which helps foster animal liberation crusades, intolerance toward opposing views, and an adversarial approach to discussion of issues like experimentation on animals.

The second reason for writing this is that I believe much of the attention and energy committed to improving the lot of animals would be put to better use ameliorating human need and suffering and in fact constitutes a diversion from this more important and indeed critical task. Now it may be replied that, of course, everyone *could* devote more time and energy to helping those who are less privileged. If we add that everyone *should* do so, then the logical extreme of this position is that anyone who fails to give up everything else he or she might otherwise be doing, including getting eight hours of sleep at night, is guilty of not putting forth enough effort to improve the lot of humankind! This is an absurd view which no one would want to endorse. My point is not that everyone should work twenty-four hours a day to improve human welfare or that everyone should work full time for a charitable or human rights organization such as Oxfam, the Foster Parents Plan, or Amnesty International, which would plainly lead to equally absurd consequences. Rather, it is that human welfare is a more vital concern than animal welfare and deserves more of our dedication because humans are more important than animals. Relieving human need and suffering is an extremely urgent priority without which our species—and indeed the natural world as such—may not survive the century. Relative to this cause, that of animal welfare, though not unimportant, appears of considerably lower priority. Lamentably, it often seems that among the most vociferous proponents of animal welfare there is an abundance of concern for the plight of other species and very little for that of our own.

Major Advances Achieved

Anyone who has looked into the matter can scarcely deny that major advances in medicine have been achieved through basic research with animals. Among these are the development of virtually all modern vaccines against infectious diseases, the invention of surgical approaches to eye disorders, bone and joint injuries and heart disease, the discovery of insulin and other hormones and the testing of all new drugs and antibiotics.

Frederick A. King, *Psychology Today*, September 1984.

In the modern era (and particularly in the nineteenth and twentieth centuries), those who object on moral grounds to the traditional ways in which nonhuman creatures have been made to serve humans have tended to adopt one of two viewpoints. The first of these is that any use of animals as means to human ends must be defended or argued for, its moral acceptability demonstrated. This position is based on the standing presumption that it is prima facie wrong to put animals to human use at all, which itself derives from fundamental convictions of the following sort: "Animals have a right to live and to be free from interference"; "Animals are sacred"; "Animals' lives are of intrinsic value, just like all of nature"; "Animals have interests that deserve equal consideration." Proponents of this view argue that any use of animals must be morally justified and often express their orientation in the idiom of rights; for example, "What *right* do we have to use animals for experimentation (even if no pain is involved)?" "What *entitles* us to interfere with the natural course of animals' lives so that we may obtain knowledge (or whatever)?" This kind of thinking lies behind the following remark by Brigid Brophy: "That I like the flavour of mutton no more entitles me to kill a sheep than a taste for roast leg of human would entitle me to kill you."

To answer the foregoing questions in their own terms would, in a way, be to share in a misconception, both of our relation to animals and of what is fundamentally at issue ethically concerning the uses to which animals are put. As I argue, the fundamental reason why we are "entitled" to use animals for experimentation—if we are forced to speak this way—is that they are in no sense the moral equals of humans, and therefore we are under no moral obligation to refrain from so using them. Since anything that is not prohibited by a moral imperative of some kind (that is, not morally wrong) is morally permissible, and since the use of animals for experimentation is not morally prohibited, then this use falls within that class of actions that are morally permissible. We do not need a correlative right to give the seal of approval to everything we do, to "justify" it. Animal liberationists frequently talk as if we do to show, allegedly, how shameful our normal practices are. But if we have no obligation toward animals to refrain from using them, as in experimentation, then we may so use them and need invoke no special entitlement, moral or otherwise, to defend this practice. The argument in favor of continuing to use animals in certain ways, then, is that the uses in question are, in and of themselves, morally neutral or morally permissible. We might indeed go beyond this and assert that animal experimentation is morally imperative or obligatory if there is no other way to obtain certain kinds of knowledge needed for the alleviation of much greater suffering in both humans and animals. . . .

Doing Harm to Animals

This difference of opinion between those who think that using animals for human ends always needs to be justified and those who do not may also stem from conflicting beliefs about whether making animals the instruments for carrying out our aims ipso facto constitutes the causing of a harm, that is, adversely affects the animals' interests (health, well-being, quality of life, and so on). . . . I do not think this is the case and that putting the matter in this way anthropomorphizes the lives of animals to an unwarranted extent. But plainly, experimenting on animals does sometimes harm them. Is this wrong? We can, if we so choose, define *harm* in such a way that injuring any sentient being—or any living thing, for that matter—is always wrong; but this would be to beg the question just posed. Some people would insist that it is always wrong (or at any rate always prima facie wrong) nonetheless. This shows, I believe, that something more basic still is at issue; namely, whether harming another creature (or life form) is a type of act that always takes place in a context of moral appraisal and which, because of this, we should uniformly judge to be wrong. Those who adhere to such a position extend what certain ethicists call the principle of nonmaleficence to animals.

Human Welfare Must Be Our Priority

Scientific inquiry into the nature of our living world has freed us from ignorance and superstition. Scientific understanding is an expression of our highest capacities—those of objective observation, interpretive reasoning, imagination and creativity. Founded on the results of basic research, often conducted with no goal other than that of increased understanding, the eventual practical use of this knowledge has led to a vastly improved well-being for humankind.

Extremists in the animal-rights movement probably will never accept such justifications for research or assurances of human treatment. They may reject any actions, no matter how conscientious, that scientists take in realistically and morally reconciling the advance of human welfare with the use of animals. But, fortunately, there are many who, while deeply and appropriately concerned for the compassionate treatment of animals, recognize that human welfare is and should be our primary concern.

Frederick A. King, *Psychology Today*, September 1984.

According to this view, it is first and foremost our duty not to harm other beings (including, of course, other humans) and only secondarily to help or benefit them (that is, to observe the principle of beneficence or benevolence). At bottom, however, this stand cannot be argued for or derived from beliefs or assumptions of a more rudimentary kind; rather, I think, it springs from a fundamental moral intuition. So the debate over the justification of animal experimentation, then, is in the final analysis over conflicting moral intuitions, neither of which is demonstrably preferable to the other. I must confess that I do not share the intuition that it is always wrong to do anything that might cause harm to an animal or that we must always have very strong and overriding reasons for doing so —especially if "harming" is taken to include (as it often is) curtailing an animal's freedom, affecting its welfare, or interfering in the normal pattern of its life in any way. For my part, it is just not self-evident that we should transfer the principle of nonmaleficence to animals. (I am assuming, for the sake

147

of argument, that it does self-evidently apply to other persons.) Nor is it even apparent that what we know of animal behavior and mental life from empirical studies should compel us to apply the principle to other species. However, this is not to say or imply that we may feel free to harm or abuse animals whenever we wish or that we lack sufficient grounds to support moral concern over animal suffering, particularly when caused by humans. Animals may not be moral agents or persons, but they may still be moral patients, that is, beings that may be affected for better or worse by our acts and which we should therefore treat with care. . . .

Reverence for Life Principle

The second prevalent moral viewpoint on our use of animals avoids the inflexibility of the position just discussed. Conceding that perhaps the human use of animals does not by itself pose a moral problem, many would still maintain that because pain is a bad thing, no matter who or what experiences it, any practice that involves inflicting suffering on sentient beings is prima facie wrong and therefore requires arguments to show why it ought not to be morally condemned. (Some would extend this claim to the taking of animal life as well, contending that a rationale must always be given to warrant such an action. Those who adhere to a Schweitzerian reverence-for-life principle, for example, would hold such a position. Others concern themselves with suffering only, allowing that killing does not pose a serious moral issue, as long as it is done painlessly or without causing undue suffering.)

This, I believe, is a much more plausible perspective and expresses a more common challenge to our present animal-use practices. For we simply do find repellent the idea of deriving benefits from suffering. . . . I argue that there are a number of confusions in the usual formulation of this position and indicate the conditions under which experimentation on animals can be justified even when it results in their suffering or death.

"Those who accept the rights view . . . will not be satisfied with anything less than the total abolition of the harmful use of animals in science."

The Case Against Animal Experimentation

Tom Regan

Tom Regan is a well-respected critic of animal experimentation. Regan believes that the use of any animal in any experiment that causes the animal mental or physical distress is morally wrong. Supporting a philosophy that he terms "the rights view," he argues that animals have the same natural rights that humans do. Whenever an animal is used in experimentation, human welfare is unfairly placed above animal welfare. In the following viewpoint, Regan presents his reasons for banning all animal experimentation. A professor of philosophy at North Carolina State University, Regan has written profusely on the topic of animal rights, including two books: *All That Dwell Therein*, and *The Case for Animal Rights*, from which this viewpoint is excerpted.

As you read, consider the following questions:

1. What is Regan's argument against using lower animals, like frogs, in experiments?
2. Why does the author believe that eliminating animal research would not seriously harm human beings?
3. Why is "the rights view" not unscientific, according to the author?

Tom Regan, *The Case for Animal Rights*. Berkeley, CA: University of California Press.

What the rights view opposes is practices that violate the basic rights of individuals in the name of "the public interest." Toxicity tests of new products that harm animals fall into this category. Anyone who objected to the rights view on the grounds that it is "morally indefensible" to release untested products into the market would miss the central point. What *is* morally indefensible is to rely on tests that violate anyone's rights. The options, then, are not *either* to continue to use these tests *or* to release untested products. A third option is *not to allow products on the market if they were pretested for toxicity on animals.* That is the option those who would dispute the rights view in the way currently under review fail to recognize. . . .

Valid Alternatives

In reply it will be claimed that no valid nonanimal alternatives exist. This is false. In the case of cosmetics, for example, the pioneering work of Beauty Without Cruelty demonstrates beyond any reasonable doubt that it is possible to manufacture and market attractive, reliable products whose toxicity for humans has not been pretested on animals. Moreover, in areas where no nonanimal tests presently exist, there is no reason why they cannot be explored, and to claim in advance that there *are none* to be found is to be guilty of being just as antiscientific as some of those who criticize animal toxicity tests. None are so blind as those who will not look. Whether found or not, whether looked for or not, the rights view's position is uncompromising: *Harmful toxicity tests of new products violate the rights of laboratory animals and ought to be stopped.* The least we, as consumers, can do to help achieve this goal is henceforth to refuse to buy any new product, including so-called, new, improved varieties of old ones, when they hit the market, unless we know that they have not been pretested for their toxicity on animals. That is a modest deprivation anyone who respects the rights of animals ought to be willing to endure.

Toxicity Tests of New Drugs

Someone might accept the preceding critique of toxicity tests on animals in the case of new products and claim that the case of doing such tests on *new therapeutic drugs* differs in morally relevant respects. No human being will be harmed in a way that is prima facie comparable to the harm caused test animals in an LD50 test, for example, by being deprived of a new brake fluid or paint. Some humans are harmed, however, right now, as a result of a variety of pathological conditions, and many more will be harmed if we fail to investigate the causes, treatments, and cures of these conditions. Indeed, some will today lose their lives as a result of these maladies, and many more will lose theirs in the future if we fail to investigate their causes and cures. Now, one thing we must do, it may be claimed, is reduce the risk that the treatment prescribed for a given malady will make patients worse-off than they otherwise would have been, and this will require establishing the toxic properties of each new drug before, not after, humans take them. Thus arises the need to test the toxicity of each new drug on test animals. If we do not test the toxicity of all new drugs on animals, humans who use these drugs will run a much greater risk of being made worse-off as a result of using them than they would if these drugs were pretested on animals. In the nature of the case, we cannot say which drugs are toxic for humans *in advance* of conducting tests on animals (if we could, there would be no need to do the test in the first place). Indeed, we cannot even eliminate all risks *after* the drug has been extensively pretested on animals (thalidomide is a tragic example). The best we can do is minimize the risks humans who use drugs face, as best we can, and that requires testing for their toxicity on animals. . . .

Humans Should Take the Risk

Anyone who elects to take a drug voluntarily chooses to run certain risks, and the risks we choose to run or, as in the case of moral patients for whom we choose, the risks we elect to allow them to run are not morally transferable to others. Coercively to harm others or to put others, whether human or animal, at risk

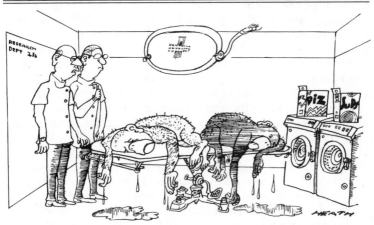

"I'm sorry they're dead, but at least it proves that one powder washes whiter than the other."

© Punch/Rothco

of harm in order to identify or minimize the risks of those who voluntarily choose to run them, is to violate the rights of the humans or animals in question. It is not *how much* the test subjects are harmed (though the greater the harm, the worse the offense). What matters is that they are coercively used to establish or minimize risks for others. To place these animals at risk of harm so that others who voluntarily choose to run certain risks, and who thus can voluntarily choose not to run them, may minimize the risks they run, is to fail to treat the test animals with that respect they are due as possessors of inherent value. . . .

A number of objections can be anticipated. One claims that there are risks and then there are risks. If we stopped testing new drugs for their toxicity, think of the risks people would run if they took them! Who could say what disastrous consequences would result? The rights view agrees. People would run greater risks if drugs were not pretested. But (a) the rights view does not oppose all pretesting (only those tests that coercively utilize some so that others may reduce those risks they may choose to run or choose not to run), and (b) those who had the choice to use an untested drug, assuming it was available, could *themselves* choose not to run the risks associated with taking it by deciding not to take it. Indeed, prudence would dictate acting in this way, except in the direst circumstances.

Four Replies to Drug Testing

Of course, if untested drugs were allowed on the market and if people acted prudently, sale of new (untested) drugs would fall off, and we can anticipate that those involved in the pharmaceutical industry, people who, in addition to their chosen vocation of serving the health needs of the public, also have an economic interest in the stability and growth of this industry, might look with disfavor on the implications of the rights view. Four brief replies must suffice in this regard. First, whatever financial losses these companies might face if they were not permitted to continue to do toxicity tests on animals carry no moral weight, since the question of overriding basic moral rights is at issue. That these companies might lose money if the rights of animals are respected is one of the risks they run. Second, there is mounting evidence that these companies could save, rather than lose, money if nonanimal tests were used. Animals are an expensive proposition. . . . Third, anyone who defends present toxicological practice *merely* by claiming that these tests are required by the involved regulatory agencies (e.g., the Food and Drug Administration) would miss the essential moral point: though these agencies have yet to recognize nonanimal tests as meeting their regulations, these agencies themselves do not require that any pharmaceutical firm manufacture any new drug. That is a moral decision each company makes on its own and for which each must bear responsibility. Fourth, appeals to what the laws require can have no moral weight if we have good reason to believe that the laws in question are unjust. And we have good reasons in the present case. Laboratory animals are not a "resource" whose moral status in the world is to serve human interests. They are themselves the subjects-of-a-life that fares better or worse for them as individuals, logically independently of any utility they may or may not have relative to the interests of others. . . .

Brutal Experiments

Academic animal research—experiments in medicine, psychology, and military testing—generally gets more publicity, partially because the details printed in professional journals are easier for the press to get hold of, but mostly because the experiments are more bizarre and alarming. Demonstrators picketed the American Museum of Natural History a while ago when word got out that experimenters there were blinding, castrating and severing the genital nerves of cats in a series of tests to determine effects on sexual behavior. Baby mice had their forelegs chopped off so that experimenters can observe whether they'll learn to groom themselves with their stumps (they learn). Baby monkeys are blinded in tests to see how fast they can find their mothers without sight (pretty fast). Electric shock is delivered to the eyelids of young mice to see how eyeshock compares in potency to footshock (too many of the test animals died in convulsions before the test could be finished). Three polar bears are submerged in a mixture of crude oil and salt water to see if they'll live (only one does). It is estimated that at least 60 million animals were "sacrificed" (the professional expression) to some kind of research in 1984 alone, many of them under conditions that can be unsentimentally described as torture.

Lillie Wilson, *The Utne Reader,* April/May 1985.

One can also anticipate charges that the rights view is antiscientific and antihumanity. This is rhetoric. The rights view is not antihuman. We, as humans, have an equal prima facie right not to be harmed, a right that the rights view seeks to illuminate and defend; but we do not have any right coercively to harm others, or to put them at risk of harm, so that we might minimize the risks we run as a result of our own voluntary decisions. That violates their rights, and that is one thing no one has a right to do. Nor is the rights view antiscientific. It places the *scientific* challenge before pharmacologists and related scientists: find scientifically valid ways that serve the public interest without violating individual rights. . . .

The rights view does not oppose using what is learned from conscientious efforts to treat a sick animal (or human) to facilitate and improve the treatment tendered other animals (or humans). In *this* respect, the rights view raises no objection to the "many human and humane benefits" that flow from medical science and the research with which it is allied. What the rights view opposes are practices that cause intentional harm to laboratory animals (for example, by means of burns, shock, amputation, poisoning, surgery, starvation, and sensory deprivation) preparatory to "looking for something that just might yield some human or humane benefit." Whatever benefits happen to accrue from such a practice are irrelevant to assessing its tragic injustice. Lab animals are not our tasters; we are not their kings.

A Moral Smokescreen

The tired charge of being antiscientific is likely to fill the air once more. It is a moral smokescreen. The rights view is not against research on animals, if this research does not harm these animals or put them at risk of harm. It is apt to remark, however, that this objective will not be accomplished merely by ensuring that test animals are anaesthetized, or given postoperative drugs to ease their suffering, or kept in clean cages with ample food and water, and so forth. For it is not only the pain and suffering that matters—though they certainly matter—but it is the *harm* done to the animals, including the diminished welfare opportunities they endure as a result of the deprivations caused by the surgery, *and* their untimely death. It is unclear whether a *benign* use of animals in research is possible or, if possible, whether scientists could be persuaded to practice it. That being so, and given the serious risks run by relying on a steady supply of human volunteers, research should take the direction away from the use of any moral agent or patient. If nonanimal alternatives are available, they should be used; if they are not available, they should be sought. That is the moral challenge to research, given the rights view, and it is those scientists who protest that this "can't be done," in advance of the scientific commitment to try—not those who call for the exploration—who exhibit a lack of commitment to, and belief in, the scientific enterprise—who are, that is, antiscientific at the deepest level. Like Galileo's contemporaries, who would not look through the telescope because they had already convinced themselves of what they would see and thus saw no need to look, those scientists who have convinced themselves that there can't be viable scientific alternatives to the use of whole animals in research (or toxicity tests, etc.) are captives of mental habits that true science abhors.

The rights view, then, is far from being antiscientific. On the contrary, as is true in the case of toxicity tests, so also in the case of research: it calls upon scientists *to do science* as they redirect the traditional practice of their several disciplines away from reliance on "animal models" toward the development and use of nonanimal alternatives. All that the rights view prohibits is science that violates individual rights. If that means that there are some things we cannot learn, then so be it. There are also some things we cannot learn by using humans, if we respect their rights. The rights view merely requires moral consistency in this regard. . . .

Mankind's Rights

Mankind's true moral test, its fundamental test (which lies deeply buried from view), consists of its attitude towards those who are at its mercy: animals. And in this respect mankind has suffered a fundamental debacle, a debacle so fundamental that all others stem from it.

Milan Kundera, *The Unbearable Lightness of Being,* 1984.

The fundamental differences between utilitarianism and the rights view are never more apparent than in the case of the use of animals in science. For the utilitarian, whether the harm done to animals in pursuit of scientific ends is justified depends on the balance of the aggregated consequences for all those affected by the outcome. If the consequences that result from harming animals would produce the best aggregate balance of good over evil, then harmful experimentation is obligatory. If the resulting consequences would be at least as good as what are otherwise obtainable, then harmful experimentation is permissible. Only if harmful experimentation would produce less than the best consequences would it be wrong. For a utilitarian to oppose or support harmful experimentation on animals, therefore, requires that he have the relevant facts—who will be benefited or harmed, how much, and so on. . . . For utilitarians, such *side effects count.* The animals used in the test have no privileged moral status. Their interests must be taken into account, to be sure, but not any more than anybody else's interests. . . .

The rights view takes a very different stand. No one, whether human or animal, is ever to be treated as if she were a mere receptacle, or as if her value were reducible to her possible utility for others. We are, that is, never to harm the individual merely on the grounds that this will or just might produce "the best" aggregate consequences. To do so is to violate the rights of the individual. That is why the harm done to animals in pursuit of scientific purposes is wrong. The benefits derived are real enough; but some gains are ill-gotten, and all gains are ill-gotten when secured unjustly.

So it is that the rights view issues its challenge to those who do science: advance knowledge, work for the general welfare, but not by allowing practices that violate the rights of the individual. These are, one might say, the terms of the new contract between science and society, a contract that, however belatedly, now contains the signature of those who speak for the rights of animals. *Those who accept the rights view, and who sign for animals, will not be satisfied with anything less than the total abolition of the harmful use of animals in science—in education, in toxicity testing, in basic research.* But the rights view plays no favorites. No scientific practice that violates human rights, whether the humans be moral agents or moral patients, is acceptable. And the same applies to those humans who, for reasons analogous to those advanced . . . in regard to nonhumans, should be given the benefit of the doubt about having rights because of the weight of our ignorance—the newly born and the soon-to-be born. Those who accept the rights view are committed to denying any and all access to these "resources" on the part of those who do science. And we do this not because we oppose cruelty (though we do), nor because we favor kindness (though we do), but because justice requires nothing less. . . .

Conclusion

To harm animals on the chance that something beneficial for others might be discovered is to treat these animals as if their value were reducible to their possible utility relative to the interests of others, and to do this, not to a few, but to many millions of animals is to treat the affected animals as if they were a renewable resource—renewable because replacement without any wrong having been done, and a resource because their value is assumed to be a function of their possible utility relative to the interests of others. *The rights view abhors the harmful use of animals in research and calls for its total elimination.* Because animals have a kind of value that is not the same as, is not reducible to, and is incommensurate with their having utility relative to the interests of others, because they are owed treatment respectful of their value as a matter of strict justice, and because the routine use of laboratory animals in research fails to treat these animals with the respect they are due, their use in research is wrong because unjust. The laudatory achievements of science, including the many genuine benefits obtained for both humans and animals, do not justify the unjust means used to secure them. As in other cases, so in the present one, the rights view does not call for the cessation of scientific research. Such research should go on—but not at the expense of laboratory animals. The overarching challenge of scientific research is the same as the similar challenge for toxicology and all other facets of the scientific enterprise: to do science without violating anyone's rights, be they human or animal.

156

"Today the idea that humans are inherently superior to the other animals rings more of self-assuring prejudice than of rational conclusion."

Animals Rights May Take Precedence Over Human Needs

Lawrence Finsen

In the battle over animal rights, animal liberationists are perhaps the most visible proponents. National newspapers frequently report their attention-grabbing methods of breaking into laboratories and hospitals and "freeing" animals from their cages. While their illegal actions are considered radical by most, Lawrence Finsen concludes that their cause is not. In the following viewpoint, Finsen argues that unnecessary and wasteful animal experimentation necessitates taking the animal rights cause seriously. He is an associate professor of philosophy at the University of Redlands in California.

As you read, consider the following questions:

1. What percentage of animal research does the author believe is valuable?
2. Why should humans care about animal suffering, according to the author?

Lawrence Finsen, "The Animal-Rights People May Not Be So 'Misguided' After All," *Los Angeles Times*, June 3, 1985. Reprinted with the author's permission.

The Animal Liberation Front raided the laboratories at UC Riverside, taking hundreds of animals and damaging property. University research projects were set back months, even years in some cases. Commentators—referring to the group's actions as "terrorist," "misguided" or the work of "demented" individuals who don't care about people—have failed to look beyond these facts.

The argument that animals should not be used in research is usually countered with the argument that human health needs take precedence over animals' rights. Many people appear relieved to have the "experts" settle the moral question in this way. They shouldn't, because the experts' argument is a distortion of the truth: Of the 60 million animals used in U.S. labs each year, only a small portion are involved in research into dread diseases such as cancer. Millions of animals die for such frivolous reasons as the testing of new cosmetics, shampoos, household cleansers and radiator fluid when safe products already exist.

The Defense Department's experiments using animals to research flesh wounds are only the most visible "use" to which the military has creatively put animals. Radiation experiments have been mutilating animals for years.

Illogical Research

Even some research aimed at promoting human health is illogical. Although we have known for some time that smoking is a health hazard, we continue to subject animals to forced-inhalation studies. The use of animals in psychological research often warrants the criticism that it receives. Researchers have been nothing less than ingenious in discovering brutal ways to model human depression, aggression and various kinds of deprivation in their animal subjects.

While much that happens to animals in labs may be innocuous, a great deal is not. Science, as a whole, is neither inherently good nor inherently evil. We must resist the tempting oversimplification implicit in defending or condemning all uses of animals with a single gesture.

A Common Assumption

Should any of this matter? Aren't humans more important than animals? The superiority of humans has been the common assumption. In an earlier, pre-Darwinian, age the clear separation of humans and others animals seemed evident. At that time the Cartesian view that we possessed souls and therefore thoughts and feelings, while no other animals did, may have been

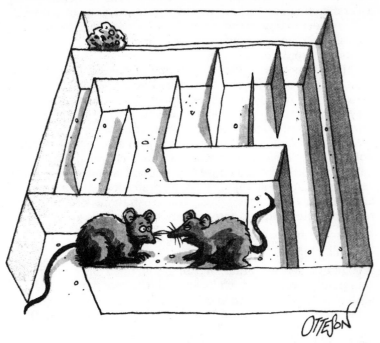

"Sure it looks easy! But if you get to the cheese, they try to give you cancer!"

reasonable. But today this view does not stand up to scrutiny. It is especially ironic that a great deal of research (such as pain studies and much psychological research) depends on the *closeness* of humans and animals rather than the reverse. There is more continuity between species than we previously thought, including the capacity to experience and suffer. Today the idea that humans are inherently superior to the other animals rings more of self-assuring prejudice than of rational conclusion. We are thus heirs to a morality that excludes serious consideration of animals' interests without benefit of adequate rationale.

Many people today are asking if the interests of non-humans do matter after all. If animals can suffer, if they have interests in living their own lives, we must ask what right we have to interfere, to impose suffering on them.

Once we view our place in the world in this light, the "need" to make animals suffer and die for our benefit is no longer so obvious. That is not to say that nothing could ever justify us in imposing suffering or killing on an animal; even human rights are not absolute. It does mean that we must provide very strong reasons to justify it, much stronger reasons than the unconvincing assurance that researchers wouldn't let their animals suffer, or the reminder that we stand to benefit from research. When viewed in this light, most of our use of animals begins to look like exploitation on a mass scale.

This does not mean that the Animal Liberation Front did the right thing by breaking into those labs, but not because its act was "lawless" or "misguided." Under certain conditions violating laws may be justifiable. We should not assume that morality must always succumb to the legal protection of institutionalized evils. We live in a world that exploits animals on an enormous scale—not just for research but also for food, clothing, sports and entertainment—and the entire force of law is on the side of the exploitation. Animals enjoy almost no protection of their interests, and certainly no legal rights. The frustrations of those who recognize the profound wrong done to animals is great indeed.

Share the Responsibility

But violating laws to appeal to the conscience of a community is a rather delicate affair. It can be justified only when that community already has significant sympathy for the lawbreakers' ideal of justice. The question of animal rights is only just beginning to be recognized as a legitimate and pressing moral question. Other avenues for change—including education, legislation and reform from within the scientific community—certainly have not been exhausted. Much more public education about the treatment of animals and their place in our moral sphere has to occur before a clear case can be made for justifying conscientious acts of resistance. But we also must remember that patience with great evil can be demanded only if real progress is possible by other means. Those who would condemn the Animal Liberation Front's actions should share the responsibility of helping to bring about significant changes to improve the lot of animals in laboratories.

"Human beings are a distinct part of nature and often must make use of the rest of nature for their own benefit, even pleasure."

Animal Rights Should Not Take Precedence Over Human Needs

Tibor R. Machan

Tibor R. Machan is a distinguished visiting professor at the University of San Diego. In the following viewpoint, Machan believes that animal liberationists go too far when they claim that animals have similar rights to life and freedom as humans. He argues that it is obvious that humans and animals are different, and that admitting this does not preclude our moral obligation to treat them humanely.

As you read, consider the following questions:

1. What crucial differences does the author see between animals and humans?
2. What absurd example does the author use to make his point that animals cannot be treated as humans?
3. What is Machan's conclusion?

"Do Animals Have Rights?" by Tibor R. Machan, first appeared in the September 30, 1985 issue of *The New American* (Belmont, Massachusetts 02178) and is reprinted by permission of the publisher. All rights reserved.

Do animals have rights similar to those we as human beings are said to have? If animals do have such rights, then by implication the government is responsible for protecting them from being killed, assaulted, or used against their will. Even the utilitarian support for what has become known as animal liberation leads to similar practical implications. If animal liberation is called for, the logical implication is vegetarianism and anti-vivisectionism for humans.

It is crucial to note that what we are addressing is not simply kindness to animals, nor that animals should be treated with consideration because of their capacity to feel pain. The kinds of stories, even movies, usually employed to buttress the case for animal liberation tend to paint a horrid picture of the pains inflicted on animals by humans. Of course, it is not entirely clear just what animals do feel; so much of what we are told and shown gains its impact in part from our awareness of how we would feel in similar circumstances. But there is little doubt that animals can feel both pain and pleasure, and that some of what human beings do to them causes great displeasure and even excruciating pain.

Too Radical

Whether treating animals shabbily is right or wrong, and what should be done about it are concerns of the animal liberation movement. But that movement has far more radical aims than improvement of the ways we handle the animals which we use for food, for medical research, and for sports. The animal liberation movement holds that animals are no different from humans in any respect, and they should not be treated differently by us—except, of course, that they cannot speak out in their own behalf or protect themselves against us. Yet, self-protection turns out to be a crucial exception. Because animals cannot defend themselves, they depend in part on us for their protection. It is indeed here that one begins to appreciate why the animal liberation movement is not, as it claims to be, analogous to the liberation of black slaves or women.

Let us be clear about this. Animal liberationists do, in fact, claim that their movement is just a logical extention of the black and women's liberation movements. Why? It is important to realize that they are convinced that there are no significant differences between animals and humans.

A moral viewpoint requires a concern for what we ought to do, not just what is good and bad. An individual could well have a theory of good and bad but still no idea what he or she ought to do, since moral obligation is also concerned with our freedom to choose. This is why the matter of free will is crucial for this debate.

It is interesting that the animal liberation movement falters exactly where it needs to take its most definite stand—whether or not animals are every bit as sovereign a part of nature as human beings. The justification for human sovereignty is our capacity to choose a line of conduct, as well as the responsibility to choose it properly. To put a proper rein on such choices, we identify certain rights and establish legal means for protecting them.

Animals Are Different

However, animals do not possess free will and thus are not faced with the moral task of choosing their conduct well. Therefore, the same claims cannot be made for them. For a being to have rights, to deserve liberation in other words, it must be able to exercise these rights and the liberty to choose. Animals would have no use for these rights, not in the sense in which humans do.

Some human beings also lack free will and moral responsibility—very young children, those in a coma, the senile, or the retarded. These last are even less easily seen as able to make use of any human rights, although some would say the same about children as well.

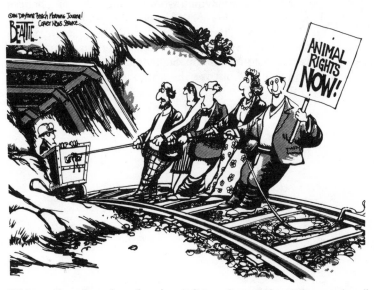

"We're putting miners down the mine shaft to make sure it's safe for canaries..."

Reprinted with permission.

Nevertheless, the position of these human beings is different from that of animals. A child is, of course, only a young human being and thus at the beginning point for complete personhood. The matter is not easy to sort out but neither is it difficult to see that children are not the equivalent of animals. With the senile and retarded we actually understand that they lack certain rights of full personhood only because of some biological imbalance, not because of their nature.

There are many problems associated with any plan to elevate animals to the equal of persons, with the rights and freedom of human beings. For example, animals kill each other, sometimes even when they belong to the same species, and it would be absurd to charge them with murder. Would animal rights require that they be prosecuted in a court of law?

Human beings should be more aware of the feelings of fellow sentient beings. Failure to do so indicates a lack of compassion and sensitivity. But compassion is one thing, animal liberation another. Human beings are a distinct part of nature and often must make use of the rest of nature for their own benefit, even pleasure.

Dangerous Hypocrisy

More likely, people will continue to entertain a schizophrenic outlook. They will both seek their own well-being and pleasure, even happiness, and at the same time feel guilty about it, and lend their support to movements which would extinguish their chances for happiness on earth. This sort of hypocrisy can be dangerous.

It would be much better to admit proudly that we value ourselves more than non-rational animals, and then extend them reasonable care and consideration. Such an attitude would, I think, be best not only for us but for the animals concerned.

Recognizing Deceptive Arguments

People who feel strongly about an issue use many techniques to persuade others to agree with them. Some of these techniques appeal to the intellect, some to the emotions. Many of them distract the reader or listener from the real issues.

Below are listed a few common examples of argumentation tactics. Most of them can be used either to advance an argument in an honest, reasonable way or to deceive or distract from the real issues. When evaluating an argument, it is important for a reader to recognize the distracting, or deceptive, appeals being used. Here are a few common ones:

   a. *bandwagon*—the idea that "everybody" does this or believes this

   b. *scare tactics*—the threat that if you don't do this or don't believe this, something terrible will happen

   c. *strawperson*—distorting or exaggerating an opponent's ideas to made one's own seem stronger

   d. *personal attack*—criticizing an opponent *personally* instead of rationally debating his or her ideas

   e. *testimonial*—quoting or paraphrasing an authority or celebrity to support one's own viewpoint

   f. *deductive reasoning*—the idea that since a and b are true, c is also true

   g. *slanters*—to persuade through inflamatory and exaggerated language instead of reason

   h. *generalizations*—using statistics or facts to generalize about a population, place, or idea

The following activity will help to sharpen your skills in recognizing deceptive reasoning. Most of the statements below are taken from the viewpoints in this chapter. *Beside each one, mark the letter of the type of deceptive appeal being used. More than one type of tactic may be applicable. If you believe the statement is not any of the listed appeals, write N.*

165

1. Millions of animals die for such frivolous reasons as the testing of new cosmetics, shampoos, household cleansers, and radiator fluid when safe products already exist.

2. Of the 60 million animals used in US labs each year, only a small portion are involved in research into dreaded diseases such as cancer.

3. All animal liberationists do, ridiculously, claim that their movement is just a logical extension of the more serious and legitimate black and women's liberation movements.

4. If animals have rights similar to those of human beings, then by implication, the government is responsible for protecting them from being killed, assaulted, or used against their will.

5. Media attention everywhere is, as always, easily and frequently captured by emotional appeals on behalf of animals and by sensationalistic tactics like "guerilla" raids on scientific laboratories "liberating" experimental animals.

6. Responsible members of the "animal rights" movement have condemned acts of violence and vandalism.

7. Human beings have believed for thousands of years that animals are *not* our moral equals, and therefore, there is no compelling ground for treating them as such.

8. Animals are in no sense the moral equals of humans, and therefore we are under no moral obligation to refrain from using them for experiments.

9. Some people today will lose their lives, and many more will lose theirs in the future, if we fail to investigate causes and cures by testing on animals.

10. Laboratory animals, to borrow a phrase from Harvard philosopher Robert Mozick, "are distinct individuals who are not resources for others."

11. If we stopped testing new drugs for toxicity on animals, think of the risks people would run if they took them! Who could say what disastrous consequences would result!

12. Scientists who protest that there are no nonanimal alternatives for experiments, in advance of the scientific commitment to try—are antiscientific.

Periodical Bibliography

The following list of periodical articles deals with the subject matter of this chapter.

The Animal's Agenda	An animal rights magazine. All issues. Available from P.O. Box 5234, Westport, CT 06881.
Ronald Bailey	"Non-Human Rights," *Commentary*, October 1985.
Stephen Begley	"Liberation in the Labs," *Newsweek*, August 27, 1984.
Lloyd Billingsley	"Save the Beasts, Not the Children?" *Eternity*, February 1985.
John R. Boyce with Christopher Lutes	"Animal Rights: How Much Pain Is a Cure Worth?" *Christianity Today*, September 6, 1985.
Matt Cartmill	"Animal Rights and Wrongs," *Natural History*, July 1986.
D. Caroline Coile and Neal E. Miller	"How Radical Animal Activists Try To Mislead Humane People," *American Psychologist* 39, June 1984.
Lisa Krieger	"Animal Use Can Be Reduced, But Not Eliminated," *American Medical News*, February 14, 1986.
National Forum	Special issue on "Animals in Society," Winter 1986.
Nature	"Opinion: Animal Rights Nonsense," vol. 305, no. 13, October 1983.
Andrew Rowan	"Why Scientists Should Seek Alternatives to Animal Use," *Technology Review*, May/June 1986.
Peter Singer	"Ten Years of Animal Liberation, *The New York Review of Books*, January 17, 1985.
Christine Stevens	"Mistreatment of Laboratory Animals Endangers Biomedical Research," *Nature*, September 1984.
Jerrold Tannenbaum and Andrew N. Rowan	"Rethinking the Morality of Animal Research," *Hastings Center Report*, October 1985.
Lee Torrey	"The Agony of Primate Research," *Science Digest*, May 1984.

What Ethical Standards Should Guide the Health Care System?

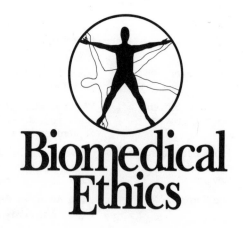

Biomedical
Ethics

"The profit-making institution in health care
[is] a moral and socially useful part of our
society."

The Profit Motive
Improves Health Care

L. John Wilkerson

Many people believe that health care should be untouched by the
profit motive; the desire to "make a buck" seems immoral and
out of place in the healing profession. However, hospitals and
physicians, faced with increasing insurance costs and enormous
malpractice awards, are more concerned than ever with making
money. In the following viewpoint, L. John Wilkerson explains
why he thinks an emphasis on profits will improve America's
health care system. Wilkerson is president of Channing, Weinberg
& Co., Inc., a health-care consulting firm in New York.

As you read, consider the following questions:

1. How does Wilkerson characterize medicine?
2. According to Wilkerson, how do not-for-profit hospitals
   compare to for-profit hospitals?
3. How does the author refute the moral argument against
   profits in health care?

L. John Wilkerson, "There Is Room for Profit in Medicine," *Los Angeles Times*, March
21, 1985. Reprinted by permission of the author.

Whatever the final fate of artificial-heart recipients William Schroeder and Murray Haydon, the reaction to the experiment has uncovered a vast store of prejudice in this country. The general target of this prejudice has been the idea of profiting from the care of the sick. The specific target has been the Humana hospital chain, which is paying the entire bill for Schroeder's treatment at the Humana Heart Institute International in Louisville, Ky.

Reasons given for criticizing Humana range all over the spectrum, but have little logical connection. Humana is accused of making this contribution as an advertising ploy to improve its image. Even if true, didn't this motive play a role in the philanthropy of the Rockefellers, the Carnegies and the like—philanthropies that still continue to contribute to society? And who is so naive to believe that there is no ulterior motive to that happy holiday tradition, Macy's Thanksgiving parade? Then Humana is accused of making its profits by refusing to give free care to the poor. In fact, most for-profit hospitals provide an amount equal to 3½% to 4% of gross revenues for free care each year.

Profit Is Not Immoral

What is most relevant in this litany of complaints is the belief by many people, including many doctors, that to profit from institutional health care is somehow immoral, that profiting from the sick is preying on the helpless—though it is not immoral to profit from selling autos or liquor or newspapers or what have you to the helpless poor. No one, not even the moralizing physicians, makes the point that a part of the relatively high fees that physicians collect is profit, just as is a part of every dollar that Humana charges.

Medicine is a business, and much of the outstanding advancement of recent years has flowed from the profit potential of contributing to earlier and superior diagnosis and therapy. Eleemosynary medicine has benefits, but they don't include the creativity and vitality that distinguish the U.S. health-care system.

What needs to be stated is the case for the profit-making institution in health care as a moral and socially useful part of our society. The first part of that case is to note that many nonprofit health-care institutions of our society are nonprofit only in theory. They often do make a profit, but at the end of the year they call it "addition to reserves" or some similar phrase.

The need to show a return on investment forces those running for-profit hospitals to focus on efficiency, on using resources creatively to most economically serve patients' needs. Since managements of for-profit hospitals get rewarded in proportion to the profit that they make, they have no inclination to tolerate the sloppy strategies and inefficiencies that often are the result of the different managerial incentives found in not-for-profit hospitals.

In for-profit hospitals, proposed capital expenditures must be measured against the likelihood that they will bring in more money than they cost, whether the expenditure is for a building or for a sophisticated diagnostic machine costing millions. Anyone who has studied nonprofit hospitals knows of numerous examples of white elephants—costly facilities or machines that lie unused or only partly used, testimony to the failure to apply tough socioeconomic analysis to the decision involved. . . .

Applying Economic Laws

The economic laws of supply and demand and competition in the marketplace apply to medicine as they do to other economic activity. . . . The profession cannot escape the economic precepts of supply and demand and market price, but economics and medicine do not need to be on opposing paths. Both are concerned about the allocation of scarce resources to increase health.

Rita Ricardo-Campbell, address to the California Society of Nursing Administrators, February 5, 1986.

But even if one accepts the economic case for profit-seeking health-care institutions—that they provide good and economical care—the moral argument still intrudes: Why should anybody profit from somebody else's misfortune?

Taken literally, this view would require that everybody involved in the health system contribute his or her services. This would mean an end to fees or salaries for physicians, nurses, hospital cleaning personnel, research scientists, workers who produce pharmaceuticals and, yes, people who write articles or books on medicine or medical care.

Why target medicine? No one objects that the farmer, food processor and grocer make a profit from the food business, yet for most people food is much more essential to their daily lives than medical care is.

A Legitimate Cost

Profit, we must not forget, is a legitimate cost of doing business in our society. Why, then, object to the role of profit in medical care, especially when—as the complex therapy given to artificial-heart recipients has shown—for-profit hospitals are increasingly providing leadership and delivering highly expert and highly humane care even for those most desperately ill?

171

"American physicians as a whole have been turned away from the ideals of service by an idolatry of money."

The Profit Motive Harms Health Care

David Hilfiker

Dr. David Hilfiker has practiced medicine in rural Minnesota and Washington, DC. He is the author of *Healing the Wounds: A Physician Looks at His Work.* In the following viewpoint, Hilfiker laments the changes in health care caused by the profit motive. Physicians, he says, have been "seduced by money," and are no longer offering the quality of care patients have a right to expect.

As you read, consider the following questions:

1. According to Dr. Hilfiker, physicians have succumbed to the profit motive "just as if we were in any other business." Why does he think this "seduction" is more disastrous in the healing profession than in other professions?
2. What are some of the dilemmas Hilfiker faces in treating patients who need "good advice" more than they need a medical procedure?
3. Do you think it is possible to be the kind of compas sionate, self-sacrificing physician Hilfiker describes? Is it prudent?

David Hilfiker, "A Doctor's View of Modern Medicine," *The New York Times Magazine,* February 23, 1986. Copyright © 1986 by The New York Times Company. Reprinted by permission.

Private medicine is abandoning the poor. As a family doctor practicing in the inner city of Washington, I am embarrassed by my profession's increasing refusal to care for the indigent; I am angry that the poor are shuttled to inferior public clinics and hospitals for their medical care. . . .

There are, of course, many complex factors that have precipitated private medicine's abandonment of the poor. The urbanization and anonymity of the poor, the increasingly technological nature of medicine and the bureaucratic capriciousness of public medical assistance—all these serve to make private physicians feel less responsible for the medical needs of those who cannot afford the going rate.

Idolatry of Money

But the cause that is probably most obvious to the lay public is singularly invisible to the medical community: Medicine is less and less rooted in service and more and more based in money. With many wonderful exceptions all over the country, American physicians as a whole have been turned away from the ideals of service by an idolatry of money. Physicians are too seldom servants and too often entrepreneurs. A profitable practice has become primary. The change has been so dramatic and so far-reaching that most of us do not even recognize that a transformation has taken place, that there might be an alternative. We simply take it for granted that economic factors will be primary even for the physician.

I do not mean merely to accuse my profession of greediness, though greed exists among doctors as among any other group. Rather, I would suggest that we physicians have been seduced by money; we have been bound by it. Money has become the measure of what we do, the yardstick of our work. Just as if we were in any other business, we physicians have capitulated to the use of economic worth as the determinant of value. In a consumer society such as ours, we doctors are not alone in our idolatry, but our seduction is such a major change from the roots of our profession that it should not go unnoticed. . . .

While we physicians have been unable or unwilling to recognize this increasing monetization of our work, society seems to have perceived it clearly and responded in kind. There are certainly many reasons for the drastic increase in malpractice judgments, but one of them is that patients are angry over the high fees physicians charge. Insurance companies recognize that patients generally sue physicians who are perceived as unsympathetic. As physicians have become wealthier, malpractice suits have risen alarmingly, and the insurance premiums have kept pace. Malpractice insurance for some specialties is now well over $50,000 a year. . . .

As the medical ethicist Albert R. Jonsen has pointed out, there has always been a tension between the Greek Hippocratic tradition and the monastic medical tradition. For the ancient Greeks, "medicine is a skill so rare that it can be sold at great price," Jonsen wrote. "It is acquired with effort, and it promises rewards." In the monastic tradition, on the other hand, monks and nuns were the healers, and "the imperatives of self-sacrifice under which they lived were extended to their duties toward the sick and dying." So the conflict is not new. What is new is the degree to which medicine has accepted the business, corporate model of measuring itself. What is new, too, I think, is the abandonment of the monastic model as idealistic nonsense.

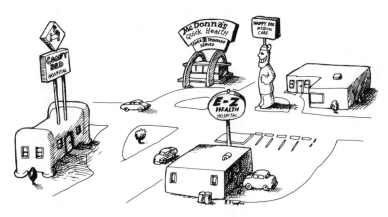

From *Dollars & Sense*, One Summer Street, Somerville, MA 02134. Reprinted with permission.

We physicians have not, I think, deliberately chosen to abandon the poor; rather, we have been blinded to our calling by the materialism of our culture and by the way medicine is structured. Many of us entered medicine out of deep altruism, wanting to be of service, only to discover that the daily crush of dozens of sick and needy souls left us exhausted. Under such circumstances, we found ways to detach ourselves from the emotional turmoil of the sick. We may have become physicians desiring to enter deeply into our patients' lives, but we soon discovered that the long lines of patients waiting to be seen encouraged us to be more "efficient" and "cost effective." We discovered that the economic pressure to see 30 or more patients a day did not allow for the kinds of relationships we had envisioned. We learned, too, that our positions of expertise, power and prestige thrust us into positions of authority from which it was difficult to escape.

The structure of day-to-day medical practice alters one's perspectives. In 10 years, I have become aware of the pressures which have subtly encouraged me to measure my work according to its economic productivity and have thus distorted the physician-patient relationship. Doctors have always been busy, I suppose, but the increasing technical intensity and busyness of medical practice has led to a preoccupation with better "management" of the office. This has generally led to the hiring of additional nurses, technicians and assistants: the physician suddenly finds himself the administrator of a large staff, a task he may never have expected and for which he was probably never prepared. Many third-party payers—insurance companies, Medicaid, Medicare and so forth—will pay only for the physician's actual, direct services, and will not pay for any tasks performed by nurses or other personnel, so the physician scurries around from patient to patient, trying to do enough to pay for the office and the staff. Very soon, a business approach seems necessary just to keep afloat, and the physician has already become an entrepreneur. . . .

The Evils of Corporate Medicine

The entrance of corporate medicine into health care has exacerbated all these tendencies. Physicians are now frequently employees of a corporation which is explicitly profit-oriented. Efficiency is now not only important but mandated from above. If the physicians, as healers, do not want to measure their work by its economic production, their employers certainly do and the attitude filters inevitably down. When the corporate body dictates that the medical care needs to become more efficient in order to increase profitability, there may be discussion about how that goal may best be attained, but ultimately there is little argument about the goal itself. . . .

The realities of medical economics encourage doctors to do less and less listening to, thinking about, sympathizing with and counseling of patients—what doctors call "cognitive services." Instead, the doctor is encouraged to *act*, to employ procedures. A procedure is anything the physician does to a patient—suturing a laceration, withdrawing fluid from a swollen joint, performing a proctoscopy, removing an appendix. Charges for procedures are a labyrinth of arbitrary rates which are almost independent of the time involved, but they are universally higher than fees for talking with the patient.

None of these pressures has caused overnight changes in physician behavior, of course, but I am aware from my own experience how a doctor's perceptions gradually evolve as a result of the economic incentives. I remember realizing one morning how

175

deeply I had changed. It was toward the end of my stay in Minnesota and before I began to work for a salary. An aged patient had come in to the office and was talking about her aching feet. She not only had several very real physical problems but she was also very lonely and quite hypochondriacal. She visited me about once a month, mostly just to complain about how people ignored her and about how lousy she felt. This month, it was her feet, swollen and aching. She lifted up her dress so I could see the feet bulging out of the shoes. It was true, the feet were swollen, but they hadn't changed perceptibly in the three years I'd been seeing this patient. I had previously tried, without much success, to explain that her obesity and sedentary life style were the primary causes of the swelling, and that I didn't have any medicines that would help her.

As she continued to tell me how tired she was, I realized I wasn't listening. I was angry. What she needed was someone to sympathize with her, gently encourage her, and to make some simple suggestions that might alleviate her suffering. I knew from past experience that that kind of listening and empathetic presence would require at least half an hour, but I would only be able to charge $20 for an intermediate call, Medicare would discount the charge significantly, and my half, after overhead, would be, maybe, $8. I also knew that if I just stood up, cut the woman off by giving her a prescription for a pain medicine and scheduled her for next month, I could charge the same $20 and move into the next room where another patient was waiting with a small laceration from which I would earn about $30 in perhaps 10 minutes.

Business Transactions

As soon as I recognized what I was angry about, I was ashamed. But the truth of my feelings was nonetheless real. Over the years, I found myself valuing brief interviews over real listening, aspiration of a joint over taking a good history, removal of an appendix over counseling a distraught teen-ager. Now I was actually angry at this old woman for taking up my time with something so economically unprofitable as listening to her story. I was looking at my interactions with patients more and more as business transactions.

There is no code in the fee book for comforting the grieving family of a patient who has just died; it is difficult to charge a panicked parent for middle-of-the-night telephone reassurance. The very fact that money has become the basis of the physician-patient interaction often inhibits a patient from raising "extraneous" issues which may be vitally important to health; it may even inhibit a patient from coming to see a doctor in the first place.

"Economic constraints . . . may be depriving some patients of their right to live."

The Poor Should Have Equal Access to Health Care

Joseph Meissner

Joseph Meissner, J.D., a graduate of Harvard Law School, is director of the Urban Development Office and the Cleveland Legal Aid Society. He is also legal advisor to Senior Citizens Coalition, the Greater Cleveland Welfare Rights Organization, and Low Income People Together. In the following viewpoint, Meissner writes that poor and disabled patients should be legally assured equal access to health care. A person's income and estimated contribution to society, he states, should not be a factor in receiving adequate care.

As you read, consider the following questions:

1. What, according to Meissner, is threatening the lives of poor people? Why are the elderly and disabled particularly at risk?
2. What is "Shaw's formulation of the quality of life"? What is the author's attitude toward this formula?
3. According to Meissner, what is the responsibility of the legal profession toward the poor?

Joseph Meissner, "Legal Services and Medical Treatment for Poor People: A Need for Advocacy," *Issues in Law & Medicine*, Vol. 2, No. 1, July 1986. Reprinted by permission of the publisher. Copyright © 1986 by the National Legal Center for the Medically Dependent and Disabled, Inc.

Poor people have long faced denial or unavailability of medically necessary health care. Today, pressures generated by demographic changes, budget cutbacks, and new methods of medical "cost containment" are combining with widespread ideological justifications for denial of treatment to threaten the very lives of increasing numbers of indigent people. The danger is particularly acute for people with disabilities and older people. Because of their disability or medical condition, many of those most at risk of denial of life preserving medical treatment lack the mental or physical ability to seek out legal assistance to defend their right to care. As a result, they have traditionally been underserved by legal services and *pro bono* attorneys. There is an urgent and growing need for affirmative action programs of outreach to those threatened populations. Only through such outreach can we hope to provide adequate legal representation in order to prevent the denial of medical treatment without which thousands may die.

The Social Lottery

In a[n] . . . issue of the *Journal of the American Medical Association,* Drs. H. Tristam Engelhardt, Jr., and Michael Rie declare that those who can afford and wish comprehensive entitlement to intensive health care treatment should be able to purchase it. However, for those who lose out in what they call the "social lottery"—those who are poor—they advocate a rationing system by which intensive care would be denied when the cost is disproportionately high or the "quality of life" of those whose lives might be saved is disproportionately low. "[I]f losing at the natural and social lotteries does not *per se* vest any individual with a claim on innocent others for care, and if the goods sought are privately owned," they write, "then the fact that individuals in need do not find resources for treatment may be an unfortunate circumstance, not an unfair circumstance."

An editorial in the same issue of this journal openly calls on physicians to move away from their traditional role of making treatment decisions on the basis of what is best for their individual patients toward a role in which they act as social surrogates for the allocation of scarce resources. These calls for rationing of health care are hardly isolated. As Patricia Nornhold, R.N., M.S.N., points out:

> As hospitals continue to cut back on codes and other expensive procedures, such as dialysis, the right-to-die issue is being overshadowed by the right-to-live issue. Economic constraints imposed by DRGs and other forms of prospective payment may

be depriving some patients of their right to live. The health care system simply can't afford these patients anymore.

Concrete examples are not hard to find. For instance, the fulminations of Dr. J. Cary Grant make clear the rising threat to indigent residents of nursing homes:

> We need to stop wasting money with unjustifiable codes [cardiopulmonary resuscitations]. . . . Codes take up the valuable time of nurses, doctors, pharmacists, and respiratory therapists. A full resuscitation can easily take an hour. It better be necessary. . . . In the final analysis, the question must be asked, "What are we saving the patient for? . . . A meaningless nursing home existence on tube feedings?"

In Ohio, a major Blue Cross and Blue Shield plan recently announced its decision that, based upon economizing, it will no longer sell individual health insurance policies to insulin-dependent diabetics, dialysis patients, people with the AIDS virus, and alcoholics. People with asthma, emphysema, tuberculosis, back and spinal injuries, as well as those with a history of blackouts, loss of consciousness, or attempted suicide, will also not be eligible for coverage. Similar proposals for other insurance carriers, using AIDS victims as the opening wedge, have appeared

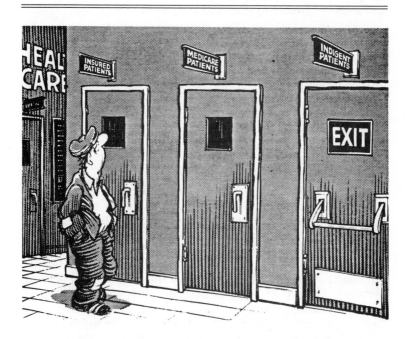

Clay Bennett for the St. Petersburg Times. Reprinted with permission.

in the media. . . .

The growing danger of denial of life-preserving medical treatment for people who are poor is particularly acute for older people and those with disabilities. Because Medicare is structured to cover the cost of treatment for acute rather than chronic illnesses and because one must "spend down" to become eligible for Medicaid, a great number of elderly persons who are significantly dependent on medical help are indigent. There is evidence that older people are more frequently denied treatment than younger ones because of a physician's presumption that social capacity declines as age advances. A study conducted at Cornell University found that physicians admitting patients more frequently suggested withholding of full medical treatment for patients over seventy-five than for younger patients with similar levels of functioning, even though age alone is not a good predictor of likelihood of survival if treatment is given. Indeed, ethicists of standing are beginning to suggest that this practice should become a formal part of public policy, as discussions at the Hastings Center demonstrate. "'[Y]ou do hear more and more quiet discussions of some sort of rationing by age, some form of triage,' Mr. Caplan [of the Hastings Center] says. Mr. Bayer agrees, adding: 'is rationing health care by age socially desirable and ethically defensible? It's an issue we're going to have to confront very soon.'''. . .

A Dangerous Trend

The American Medical Association's Council on Ethical and Judicial Affairs proclaimed that it is appropriate to withhold all life support, *including food and water*, from irreversibly comatose individuals whose death is not imminent. If that principle is extended to the next level of neurological unconsciousness, the "permanent vegetative state," it could affect 10,000 Americans whose nutrition might be cut off due to their impaired states of consciousness.

Such developments in medical practice and thought must be considered in light of our country's demographic changes. It is widely recognized that the American population is aging and that this will have severe economic and social consequences. In 1982, there were fifty-four people of working age (eighteen to sixty-four years old) for every ten over sixty-five. In the year 2025, the U.S. Census Bureau predicts that ratio will be only thirty-to-ten. . . .

It takes no crystal ball to predict that the economically induced pressures against the right of indigent older people to receive medical treatment are likely to increase, not decrease. This dangerous trend imposes special responsibilities on those who serve the legal needs of poor people. Resort to the legal process may frequently be all that stands between indigent older people and the denial of life preserving medical treatment. As surely as in criminal cases involving indigent defendants threatened with capital punishment, the availability of vigilant advocacy by competent attorneys may be the only protection for these individuals against unwarranted death sentences.

Just as those subject to discriminatory denial of medical treatment on the basis of age are disproportionately poor, so also are those in the other category most likely to be denied life-preserving medical treatment: people with disabilities. . . .

Maintaining Care for the Poor

Health care for the poor remains a critical concern. Persons without health insurance, or those relying on stingy Medicaid programs, will find their options even more limited, if they have any options at all. As hospitals scramble to join HMOs and PPOs, and as patients with copayments use fewer services, hospitals will not be generating surplus funds to help pay for money-losing care for the poor. Without government action, much of the savings resulting from these reforms will come from reducing services given to the poor and near-poor.

We can work towards a system perhaps, of competing HMOs, each with a strong consumer power. Wasteful care could be reduced, prevention and needed care encouraged. But all the pressure now is from corporations and insurance companies concerned about lowering costs. We must work to ensure that health care costs are not cut merely by cutting health care.

Sam Baker, *Diagnosis: Capitalism*, 1985.

Among the population of persons with disabilities, discriminatory denial of medical treatment specifically based on poverty has been encountered. Physicians at one state hospital explicitly justified decisions to deny life-preserving medical treatment based on the lower economic status of patient's families. In deciding to recommend the denial of treatment to nearly half (48%) of the children with spina bifida seen during a five year period, the hospital's health care team wrote,

> We have . . . been influenced by Shaw's formulation of the quality of life. In this formula, $QL = NE \times (H+S)$, QL is quality of life, NE presents the patient's natural endowment, both physical and intellectual, H is the contribution from home and family, and S is the contribution from society. . . . [T]here is no evading the fact that external circumstances are crucially important in the outlook for the newborn with myelomingocele. Thus, the treatment for babies with identical "selection criteria" could be quite different depending on the contribution from home and society. . . .

As the noted civil libertarian and *Village Voice* columnist Nat

Hentoff has written, "Since under this formula the patient's natural endowment is not the sole determinant of the medical treatment he gets, his chances of being permitted to stay alive can be greatly reduced if his parents are on the lower rungs of poverty.". . .

Devaluation of the lives of those with disabilities, often expressed in terms of pity and a paternalistic conclusion that their "quality of life" is so low that they would be better off dead, runs deep in our society. A California appellate court describes an individual with cerebral palsy as one whose "quality of . . . life has been diminished to the point of hopelessness, uselessness, unenjoyability and frustration. . . . [The] petitioner would have to be fed, cleaned, turned, bedded, toileted by others for 15 to 20 years!" Dr. George Crile writes of "society's right for its members to have pleasant and productive lives, not to be lived to support the growing numbers of hopelessly disabled, often unconscious people whose costly existence is consuming so much of the gross national product.". . .

Legal Assistance Needed

People with disabilities of all ages face discrimination in the availability and delivery of medical services. These persons are often incompetent or unconscious when critical decisions on lifesaving medical treatment must be made. Many are in nursing homes or hospitals on public assistance. When legal assistance is needed to represent their interests, they frequently do not have the resources to afford their own counsel. Legal services or *pro bono* attorneys must step forward to represent them as attorneys or as guardians ad litem.

The gathering storm clouds of financial privation, together with the growing tendency unapologetically to devalue the lives of those at the margins of our society, especially indigent people with disabilities and indigent older people, makes representation of such clients in defense of their right to receive medical treatment an increasingly urgent challenge to legal services providers. It is a challenge that can be met only by expanding our ability to take affirmative action in providing outreach to this vulnerable and underserved population, which is all too often incapable of seeking us out.

"Scarcity . . . requires that we say 'no' to some people whom we would like very much to help."

Equal Access to Health Care Is Impossible

E. Haavi Morreim

Americans have often looked on hospitals as "good samaritans," believing that the health care industry has sufficient resources to provide health care to all who need it, including those who cannot pay for it. However, according to E. Haavi Morreim, author of the following viewpoint, health care resources are not unlimited and therefore cannot be available to everyone. Though denial of health care may seem unfortunate, she says, it is not unjust. Morreim, assistant professor in the College of Medicine at the University of Tennessee in Memphis, is a philosopher and author concerned with the interaction of medicine, law, and philosophy.

As you read, consider the following questions:

1. According to Morreim, why are the cost-cutting measures taken so far by federal and state governments insufficient?
2. Describe the five proposals for allocating scarce health care resources. What, according to the author, are the shortcomings of each?
3. What does Morreim mean by "unfortunate does not mean unfair"? Do you agree? Why or why not?

E. Haavi Morreim, "Who Shall Live" was originally published in the spring 1985 issue of *Touchstone*, the magazine of the Tennessee Humanities Council. Reprinted with permission.

Health care costs in the United States have escalated enormously during the past 15 years. Health care delivery now comprises nearly 11 percent of the Gross National Product and is expected to grow by an average $50 billion per year, doubling every six years between now and the year 2000. Federal Medicare outlays for the elderly have risen by about 17 percent since 1970, and could result in a deficit of $300 billion by 1995 unless current trends are substantially altered. States' Medicaid expenditures grew by 22 percent between 1981 and 1983, nearly twice as fast as state tax revenues. And corporations, who pay one-third of the nation's health care bill through employee benefits, are likewise laboring under an escalating burden. The Chrysler Corporation, for example, spent over $400 million on health care benefits in 1984—that's $5,700 per active worker or $550 per car.

In response, the federal and state governments and the private sector have taken numerous and varied steps to curb health care cost increases, from Medicare's DRG prospective payment plan, to state-mandated caps on health care spending, to health and fitness programs for employees in the workplace. Quite likely, substantial initial savings can be garnered from cutting out the "fat" in health care services. Physicians are learning to be more careful in ordering tests, patients are seeking second surgical opinions more often, insurance companies are scrutinizing charges more closely, hospitals are joining together to purchase common items in bulk. In these ways we can economize on quantity without impairing quality.

Major Cutbacks Necessary

Unfortunately, such benign trimming probably will not be sufficient. The economic pressures necessitating cost containment are likely to worsen before they improve. The national debt has reached unprecedented proportions, requiring major cutbacks in a number of national projects; and although important, health care is not the nation's only nor even its most important spending priority. By the same token, corporations, facing an increasingly competitive international market, are anxious to curb the fringe benefits expenses which raise their production costs. Thus, although eliminating truly unnecessary practices is a start, eventually our continued need for economic cutbacks is likely to mean some reductions in both the quantity and quality of necessary care.

At the same time, pressures to continue or even increase our present levels of health care are substantial. Physicians and other providers are morally, professionally, and legally loath to abridge their fiduciary commitment to their patients in order to ease some third-party's pocketbook. And as citizens we have come to expect, even to demand, virtually unlimited access to ever-improving medical technology. We are deeply reluctant to see anyone denied vital health care for financial reasons. We are particularly distressed to see someone die who could have been saved by an existing technology if only he'd had the money to pay for it.

The Case of Hemodialysis

This was the situation in the mid-1970s, when there were too few hemodialysis units to serve all those suffering from endstage renal disease (ESRD). Those who received dialysis lived; those who didn't died. To choose among applicants in some morally defensible way, many localities established selection committees. One of the best known was the Seattle Artificial Kidney Center at Swedish Hospital in Seattle, Washington. After first eliminating on medical grounds those less likely to survive even with dialysis (e.g., people who suffered other life-threatening diseases), the committee turned to criteria of social worth, including marital status, occupation, number of dependents, church membership, and social contributions such as scout leadership.

Spending America's Limited Resources

There are *anti-social ethics* in medicine and health care. Real ethics teach us we must do more than "mean well," we must also "do good." Medical care is a drain of resources. You are spending America's limited resources. You are trustees of this nation's wealth; you hold part of the future. Health care has the ability to bankrupt America—to prevent us from meeting other important social goals. . . .

Each dollar spent on health care is a dollar that cannot be spent on something else. No set of expenditures can rise faster than the Gross National Product forever.

Richard D. Lamm, speech delivered to the American Hospital Association, February 11, 1985.

Upon reaching the public eye, such selection procedures caused considerable consternation. As observed by David Sanders and Jesse Dukeminier, Jr.: "The Pacific Northwest is no place for a Henry David Thoreau with bad kidneys." After a powerful lobbying effort, the need for such choices was eventually obviated after Congress voted in 1973 to provide full payment for the treatment of any person suffering from end-stage renal disease. Coverage now includes not only hemodialysis, but other forms of treatment such as peritoneal dialysis and kidney transplant. The total ESRD program currently costs upwards of $2 billion per year.

In 1973 we faced the terrible choices of scarcity by eliminating the scarcity. Whether or not this approach was the best way to address the ESRD situation, it is a luxury we can no longer afford. The nation's boundless scientific creativity may always find better ways to treat virtually any disease, but the needs of the ill and the costs of such new treatments are equally boundless. Consider, for example, our newfound abilities to transplant a variety of organs, including not only kidneys, but livers, lungs, pancreases, hearts, and now even artificial hearts. We cannot afford to provide every service for everyone in need, yet how shall we decide who will receive these life-saving procedures? Our present practices seem arbitrary and even unfair. Those who happen to need kidneys have financial access to every opportunity to live, while those who need a liver must die unless they can pay the enormous bills themselves. Is there some clear, morally comfortable way of resolving such questions?

Allocation Alternatives

For purposes of our discussions, let us assume that availability of organs were not a problem and that finances were our only obstacle. I would suggest that society cannot escape those terrible choices with which we wrestled, then temporarily managed to dodge, during the early days of dialysis. Let us briefly examine several different ways which have been proposed to resolve with a minimum of moral distemper. We will see that though such remedies can help, we must still in the end answer very difficult questions.

First, let us consider some financial approaches.

(1) Suppose, for example, that we tried to stretch our resources by requiring that all patients who are financially able pay their own health care expenses as far as possible. This seems socially and morally helpful, for it would enable us to help more people with society's funds. Unfortunately, this remedy will still leave us to confront difficult choices. We will still come to the end of our finite resources, and if there is not enough to help everyone, we will still be forced to choose whom we shall help and whom we shall not.

(2) As another financial approach, suppose that we establish *regional transplant centers*—designating only selected hospitals to perform all the necessary transplant operations. On the positive side, regionalization may help to avoid needless duplication of facilities and to ensure that those who perform these procedures have sufficient experience and expertise to avoid costly and sometimes tragic errors in technique or follow-up care.

Once again, however, the economy we stand to gain here is too limited. First, duplication of facilities may not be such a problem in the first place. The technical equipment required for transplant is already possessed by many hospitals. And while the acquisition of experience is indeed important, even a complete avoidance of unnecessary complications and errors will not solve our most basic allocations question: who shall be eligible to receive a transplant in the first place? . . .

Criteria of Medical Benefit

(3) Suppose that we appealed to *criteria of medical benefit* to limit the number of people to whom we offer transplant. Surely this must be at least a part of our answer, for it would be not only foolish but morally wrong to waste such precious resources on those who cannot benefit, while letting die some of those who could be saved. Thus we may rightly deny transplant to those who will die soon no matter what we do, to those who cannot survive the surgery, or to those competent patients who have conscientiously judged their own quality of life to be so marginal that they believe the added burdens of treatment would not be worthwhile.

Learning To Say No

The health-care problem is not a federal or state budget problem. It is a social problem. The expenditures are the same regardless of whether the money is spent through the federal budget or private insurance. Somehow, we have to learn to say "no."

Lester C. Thurow, *Harper's*, April 1985.

Unfortunately, such benefit criteria will not take us far. There are few people for whom life itself is not a benefit. If we wish further to appeal to "medical" criteria, we must implicitly rely on some very nonmedical values. Indeed, this is precisely what the early dialysis committees did as they screened candidates on "medical" grounds. Diabetics, for example, were routinely denied eligibility by the Seattle committee, as were children, anyone over age 45, and those with other co-morbidities such as heart disease or mental illness.

Though it is a medical judgment that these people were less likely to survive as long as the others and more likely to suffer complications, it requires a moral judgment to say that these people should be denied the opportunity for whatever life may be available to them. Their exclusion from eligibility rests on an implicit moral belief that scarce resources ought to be used, not simply for those who would benefit at all, but for those who are most sure to benefit and whose benefits would be greatest. To allow a "sure survivor" to die while supporting someone who might not survive or who would survive less long was thus considered a "waste" of resources. . . .

(4) Suppose we return to *criteria of social worth*, as the Seattle committee did after screening for "medical" eligibility. It should be immediately obvious that difficult moral decisions would be required. Even if we were able to factor out the social biases which have led us to undervalue selected groups of people on the basis of race, age, or sex, we would still have to justify morally the idea that someone's access to lifesaving resources should be based on his usefulness to the rest of us. And we would need to figure out what is to count as "useful," and why.

(5) Finally, suppose that instead we turn to a more *egalitarian approach*, distributing available organs by some random method—a lottery perhaps—which literally gives each person the same chance for help as anyone else. While this would save us from difficult choices among those who are placed in the lottery, we still cannot escape some vexing questions. Who is to be eligible for the lottery in the first place? Will we allow an alcoholic equal access to a liver transplant? Will we enter onto the list a person who had already received a transplant and who, through his own failure to adhere to medication and dietary restrictions, has caused his first organ to be rejected? Shall we admit those who have only a marginal chance to survive?

Denial Not Morally Wrong

In sum, there is no escape from making some terribly difficult choices. Scarcity, in its very essence, means that some of the people who need and deserve a resource must go without, and this in itself requires that we say "no" to some people whom we would like very much to help.

Yet the scarcity which poses this moral consternation can also offer moral consolation. Unmet needs do not imply moral wrong. Even the best allocation policies will produce unfortunate consequences, but unfortunate does not mean unfair. The morally important questions are whether our allocation policies are fair and just, and whether they achieve a reasonable amount of good. If they are, then no one can complain. No one has a right to that which is scarce, and one is not wronged in being denied what he was never owed. As a society we must recognize that we face these moral choices. We cannot label them as "medical" in order to thrust them upon health care providers, nor can we ignore them in hopes that they will go away or resolve themselves. The nation's economic constraints ensure that they will not go away, and any resolution-by-default is sure to be less fair than a carefully reasoned, publicly argued decision in which the interests of all can be heard and considered.

"Though the technology of medicine . . . may 'fix up' a broken or diseased body, a return to health demands that the patient participate in the healing process, or it doesn't work."

Health Care Should Focus on the Patient

Roger S. Jones and Lawrence LeShan

Roger S. Jones is an associate professor of physics at the University of Minnesota and the author of *Physics as Metaphor*. In Part I of the following viewpoint he writes that science has dehumanized medical care. He believes more emphasis must be placed on holistic healing. In Part II Lawrence LeShan offers a definition of holistic healing. He explains how holistic principles can improve health care by taking into account the spiritual and relationship needs of the patient. LeShan is a research psychologist and author of numerous books.

As you read, consider the following questions:

1. Why does Jones believe that people idolize science? Why is that idolatry breaking down?
2. What is LeShan's complaint with present medical technology?
3. Why is holistic healing better than a scientific or technological approach to medicine, according to LeShan?

Roger S. Jones, "We're Worshiping a Golden CAT Scan," *The Washington Post National Weekly Edition*, July 21, 1986. Reprinted with the author's permission.
From *The Mechanic and the Gardener* by Lawrence LeShan. Copyright © 1982 by Lawrence LeShan. Reprinted by permission of the author.

I

''Neuroscientists are beginning to suspect that everything that makes people human is no more than an interaction of chemicals and electricity inside the labyrinthine folds of the brain,'' said *Newsweek* on Feb. 7, 1983.

This quotation pretty well sums up the prevailing scientific attitudes about life and consciousness. At any moment we can expect an announcement that the secret of life has been discovered and that life has been created artificially in a test tube. Science has not yet accomplished this feat, but there is every reason to believe that it will before long. Genetically manufactured drugs and organ transplants are already commonplace. Now that we understand DNA, our complete control over the processes of life is only a matter of time.

Scientific Idolatry

This may sound to some like the epitome of progress, but I see it as a tragic step in our dehumanization. Not only does it portend some mechanical or chemical variety of humanity, it hastens our spiritual deterioration by strengthening what I call scientific idolatry.

Whenever we lose sight of the human source and origin of an idea, it becomes an idol—a symbol to which we attribute an absolute and objective authority. As Einstein and others have pointed out, the theories of science are fundamentally creations of the human mind. But because science claims to deal with an objective reality, we tend to treat its ideas and models as real and independent of their human creators. We idolize the concepts and theories of science.

The biblical sin of idolatry refers not just to the making of graven images, but to their worship. Idolatry in contemporary life is not as remote and anachronistic as it may seem. Neither the prophets of ancient Israel nor the medieval church fathers ever had to deal with idolatry on the vast scale that exists today in the name of science. For science has become our state religion, scientists our infallible priests, and scientific theories our icons and salvation. . . .

The Breakdown of Science

Despite the powerful hold scientific idolatry has on us, there is growing evidence of its breakdown, especially in the health sciences. It has become apparent that drugs, surgery and feats of technology have come up against major obstacles in the treatment of cancer and other degenerative diseases. The traditional medical model seems almost overwhelmed by the efforts to treat illness in purely materialistic terms.

There has been a steady increase in recent years in the use of alternative medical techniques: homeopathy, acupuncture and eastern folk and herbal medicine, spiritual healing, dietary therapies, and various psychological or psychic treatments that involve the use of imagery and meditation. All of these holistic therapies assume the cooperation of mind and body.

Dr. Karen Olness, for example, of the Children's Hospital in Minneapolis, has successfully used imaging and hypnosis in the treatment of children with terminal illnesses. Earl Bakken, the inventor of the pacemaker and president of Medtronics Corp., suggests that for purely economic reasons the growing use of high-tech medicine will have to be curtailed. Psychic and holistic techniques have become a practical necessity.

II

As a nation we spend over $250 billion a year on medical care. (Over $6 billion worth of prescriptions are written each year.) It is difficult to comprehend such figures—but one thing seems quite clear: most people don't feel it is enough. Patients complain that there are not enough doctors and nurses; doctors and nurses complain they don't have enough technicians, enough space, enough equipment. Hospitals get bigger and bigger—to such a point that it has become impossible to find one's way to a specific service without streaks of different colors along the floors or walls, and a map more complicated than those for most cross-country highways.

As a Person

You should expect your physician to deal with you as a person, not as an isolated set of symptoms, and to consider your illness as an occurrence in your individual life. You can expect him to discuss with you matters of personal habit and hygiene that may have led to the illness, and the alterations of personal habit that may help you to recover from it. Physicians as well as patients have to assume a new kind of responsibility in dealing with illness.

Paul Snyder, *Health & Human Nature*, 1980.

As in so many other spheres of life, the human need for personal attention, loving care, intimate contact hasn't changed, but everything has changed about medical services, so that while we hear daily about wonderful, thrilling new breakthroughs, medical discoveries that can save lives, most of us who need to have contact with doctors and hospitals usually feel lost, alone, confused, and anonymous. We lose our identity, we begin to feel we are nonpersons. . . .

One of the most devastating features of the advances in medical techniques and knowledge has been the tendency to identify people by disease or by organ only. There is the classic story of the surgeon who tells his office nurse, "Send in the stomach case now, I'll see the liver after that." The more we learn about the *technical craft* of saving physical life, the less we seem to have kept in touch with the *human art* of caring about the person.

Recently I visited a hospital in West Virginia where I worked thirty-eight years ago. At that time it was a 2,500-bed army medical facility constantly full of the casualties of World War II. It was a one-story building and every ward faced the open air and had grass and trees on three sides. In spite of its size it was a close-knit and caring place with a warm and friendly atmosphere. Everyone, patients and staff alike, gathered in off-hours at the central recreation area, "Times Square," with its coffee shop, lounge areas, auditorium, and movies.

The Human Art of Caring

When I came back to it this year the place was still much the same. Now a veterans' hospital, it still retained in its wards and corridors the same warm, informal, and caring atmosphere it had had in the past. The countryside was still green all around it. The patient population tended to be older, but outside of that I couldn't find too much change. I talked informally to patients and staff and received the same impression from both. It is still a hospital where, if you are a patient, you know that the staff is primarily interested in taking care of you. You feel safe and protected.

A quarter of a mile behind it a new structure is being built. This is the new hospital that in a year or so will replace the old one. It is sixteen stories high, very modern; a giant box of a place. It will be technologically more efficient than the old rambling building. However, none of the wards will have open air on three sides nor will a patient be able to get out of bed, walk ten feet, and sit on a lawn. I know from experience that the entire atmosphere and tone of the place will also change. Concern will shift from patient care to technology. Patients will be less and less the central focus of the organization and more and more business criteria and engineering concepts will take their place. The rate of patient recovery will go down. In spite of the fact that every study has shown that recovery from serious illness takes place most rapidly in an intimate and caring environment, hospitals keep getting bigger and bigger and more oriented toward modern technology. The new building will probably save some money per patient day in the long run. It will also increase the average time patients stay and will thus have a higher cost in every way when the total picture is in.

In recent years—due in good part to the lack of caring for the whole person in mainline medicine—we have seen the remarkable and rapid rise of a new medical model, which generally is described as "holistic medicine." The term has come to mean a variety of things—from nutrition to acupuncture to psychic healing—but what all holistic methods have in common is the underlying hunger, the profound search, for some way to see and respond to the patient as a complete person, not just as a collection of functioning or nonfunctioning organs.

For what we are more and more aware of is that though the technology of medicine, the bigger and bigger hospitals, and the growing depersonalization thereby created may "fix up" a broken or diseased body, a return to health demands that the patient participate in the healing process, or it doesn't work.

The present public interest in "holistic medicine" in all forms, both sensible and silly, involving both practitioners of integrity and charlatans, has developed primarily because of this awareness that technology is not enough. The exact meaning of the term, however, eludes us. New modalities of treatment constantly appear, leaving us hopeful but confused.

Ignoring the Patient's Needs

The doctor said: this-and-that indicates that this-and-that is wrong with you, but if an analysis of this-and-that does not confirm our diagnosis, we must suspect you of having this-and-that. If we assume that you have this-and-that, then . . . and so on. There was only one question Ivan Ilyich wanted answered: was his condition dangerous or not? But the doctor ignored that question as irrelevant. From the doctor's point of view, such a question was unworthy of consideration. One had only to weigh possibilities: floating kidneys, chronic catarrh, or an ailment of the caecum. There was no question of the life of Ivan Ilyich.

Leo Tolstoy, "The Death of Ivan Ilyich," 1887.

A major part of the development, however, is clear. It is concerned with widening the view of the patient; with the understanding that *all* levels of his being are of equal importance in the prevention of disease and the search for health. In the cure of disease, this wider interest also has the purpose of bringing more strongly into play that patient's own self-healing and self-repair abilities—of bringing these capabilities to the aid of the medical program. These "other" levels comprise a wide range, from the nutritional to the spiritual, and include the patient's relationship needs and creative needs.

193

"Pay attention to what the social scientists are saying about medicine, but don't let them argue you away from science."

Focusing on the Patient Is Not Enough

Lewis Thomas

Lewis Thomas, a well-known biologist and essayist, is president emeritus of the Memorial Sloan-Kettering Cancer Center. He has written several popular books on science, including *Lives of a Cell* and *Late Night Thoughts on Listening to Mahler's Ninth Symphony.* In the following viewpoint, Thomas explores the role of scientific research in health care. Ultimately, Thomas says, the key to health lies in medical science.

As you read, consider the following questions:

1. According to Thomas, what is the problem with today's medical care?
2. Why does Thomas disagree with the critics of technological science?
3. What, according to the author, is the first priority of medicine? What does he place in secondary importance?

Lewis Thomas, "Medicine Needs More Research, Not More 'Caring.'" *Discover,* September 1985. Reprinted by permission of Harold Ober Associates Incorporated. Copyright © 1985 by Lewis Thomas.

If you don't take good care of yourself these days you're risking more than your health. You could lose your standing as a decent, upright member of the social order. It's becoming a hard life to get through, even though most of us seem to be managing it, all by ourselves, and for a longer run than at any other time in man's history. Reaching into our seventies and eighties is child's play, and our wives can begin looking forward to 100 or 110 birthday candles.

Up to now we've been doing this pretty much by ourselves, occasionally tapping into what's currently known as the Health Care System, but tapping only tentatively and gingerly. We've tended to look on longevity as something that happens naturally—not entirely naturally, perhaps, considering the crucial role played over the past two centuries by good plumbing, sanitary engineering, childhood immunization, plenty of food and shelter thanks to Western-style agriculture and architecture, and, in a phrase, a better standard of living. A better standard of living is probably something rather different from Letting Nature Take Her Course, and, to be sure, there's nothing quite natural about modern medicine and surgery.

But now, I'm apprehensive to say, we're entering a new world of *advice*, and taking care of oneself is beginning to look much more complicated than it once was. Learning and mastering all the rules is itself an exhausting business and bad enough, but the hardest part of taking care of oneself is the personal sense of guilt when the rules aren't followed. There's simply no doubt at all that the rising cost of health care can't keep rising, and no doubt that it's caused by everyone overusing the Heath Care System.

What To Do?

But what is one to do? Being sick in a hospital these days is beginning to seem like an antisocial act. There you are, in a bed costing the insurance industry $750 or more a day just for the bed, and in comes the orderly to wheel you off for a CT scan or a glimpse of the tail of your pancreas under magnetic resonance imaging—and up goes the Gross National Deficit. And, if you've read the newspapers or listened to television, or even strolled past the paperback shelves in the local bookstore, you must know that you'd never have landed in the hospital in the first place if only you'd followed the rules and looked after yourself. Exercise, for example. Diet, for another. The latest Good Habit is eating fiber to prevent cancer and it's made to sound, in the commercials for breakfast cereals, more like Moral Fiber than food. It's become virtuous to be healthy and very nearly larcenous to be ill. Not long ago, I read a wonderful article about the challenges faced by any careful reader of Jane Brody's column in the *New York Times*. Brodyland, the writer called it, a world filled with advice about the avoidance of menaces to health and survival. I've read some of her columns, and what strikes me is the number of menaces that accompany simply thinking wrong. You can develop cancer, heart disease, and stroke, all three maybe at once, by acquiring the wrong sort of personality. And you shouldn't, because everyone else has to pay for it, and that'll make you feel guilty. I don't know how many other costly diseases are the result of the stress caused by feelings of guilt.

Positive Thinking Is Not Enough

Nothing is more painful to a patient dying of cancer than adding personal guilt to the disease. Yet certain scientists are now pushing the notion that how you think and feel can determine how the disease spreads. . . .

This is heartening to those of us who believe we can control . . . disease, but it does not tell us much. . . . The most reliable indicator for how a cancer grows is the biological nature of the cancer and the treatment applied. A good attitude—what Norman Vincent Peale called "the power of positive thinking" and the Rev. Robert Schuller calls "possibility thinking"—usually enhances the quality of life, but to prescribe a psychology as a way of fighting cancer is to make the patient bear the burden for his own cure.

Suzanne Fields, *The Washington Times*, November 5, 1985.

The cigarette smoker isn't just a defiant enemy of society. He's a *troubled* person in need of counsel. When you next smell the whiff of distant smoke, you should know that someone out there is really signaling for help, like the writing on the bathroom mirror: "Stop me before I smoke again!"

Preventive medicine is all over the place, warning against this or that. Only aging and dying are the insoluble problems, not to be confronted by easy aphorisms or hunches. But aphorisms do abound, some of them good. "Age dry," the French used to say, meaning, I think, get thinner and thinner until finally you turn to dust and blow away, rather like the perfectly made coach in Oliver Wendell Holmes Sr.'s famous metaphor for aging and death, the one-hoss shay.

"Aging's not for sissies," I recall someone saying.

And we have a lot still to learn. The critics of medicine are all over the place, and their voices are rising. There's too much science in medicine already, it's asserted, and it costs too much, fails to provide the benefits it's supposed to provide, and interferes too often with the old art of medicine and the "caring" functions of doctors. There's something to this criticism, of course. It's based on some of the more spectacular technologies developed just within the past decade or so for the prolongation of life—the introduction of life-support systems for patients dying of chronic, irreversible diseases; the transplantation of hearts, livers, kidneys, pancreases, lungs; and, most headline-catching of all, the invention of the artificial heart. The critics assert—and I agree with them—that no society can possibly tolerate many more such gifts from medical science, nor can any system of financing, public, private, or both, afford the costs of extending such benefits (if indeed they are benefits) to everyone needing them. But I disagree with the implied assertion that these are the right examples of where science has been taking medicine, or will be taking it.

To the contrary, in my view these technologies are, in their very existence, the best of arguments for more basic biological research. The artificial heart is here because we haven't the ghost of an idea about the pathogenesis of the heart disease called cardiomyopathy (which will almost certainly turn out to be a virus infection), and it will still be with us, causing an increasingly intolerable burden of cost, for as long as we remain ignorant of the underlying causes of this and other forms of heart failure—including, in the years just ahead, the commonest of all: coronary heart disease. Unless we learn the real, central causes of coronary occlusion, and then learn how to prevent it, the artificial heart will be in production out there, costing the moon and impossible to prohibit.

We're obliged to use kidney transplantation and chronic renal dialysis because we don't really understand the mechanisms of chronic glomerulonephritis and pyelonephritis, two causes of kidney failure, and we're therefore unable to cure these diseases in their early stages, or to prevent them.

The Record of Biomedical Science

You'll hear it argued that we can't rely on the past record of biomedical science to forecast the future, because the diseases now on the agenda are fundamentally different in nature. To be sure, it's conceded in this argument, medicine has transformed the treatment and prevention of infectious disease, so that we no longer see the wards of city hospitals filled, as they were during my internship, with patients dying of lobar pneumonia or miliary tuberculosis or septicemia or acute rheumatic carditis or tertiary syphilis. But it's said, those were different kinds of disease, with a single cause that could be got at.

Today's health problems are of quite a different order, it's claimed: they're chronic illnesses, for the most part affecting the elderly—chronic heart failure, arthritis, diabetes, senile dementia, cancers of a hundred different kinds, strokes and things of that nature. Moreover, it's said, they probably don't have single causes and there's no use in doing research that looks for single causes: they're "multifactorial," as the trendy term has it. They're even said to be societal in orgin. I don't believe any of this. The assertion that today's chronic diseases—rheumatoid arthritis, for example—are multifactorial and therefore far beyond scientific reach, is simply another way of saying that we're still too ignorant about the mechanisms of disease.

The Triumphs of Science

Never in all of history has medical science made life so long or so free of disease. . . .

"We live in an era when some dramatic new development is reported every day," says Dr. Frederick Robbins, former president of the Institute of Medicine in Washington, D.C. . . . "We should eventually be able to develop safe, effective tools to combat any organism that causes disease."

Abigail Trafford, *U.S. News & World Report*, November 11, 1985.

But the future is out there, somewhere ahead, and it's a scientific future. Medicine is still a relatively ignorant profession, with a great deal yet to be learned, but it's at last clear that the learning can be done, the mechanisms of disease can be looked for by the methods of science, and sooner or later, depending on how hard the investigators in our youngest generation work and how lucky they are, we'll do as neat a job on schizophrenia and Alzheimer's disease as an earlier generation did on general paresis and tabes dorsalis—respectively, paralysis and spinal cord degeneration resulting from syphilis. Be kind to our friends the psychoanalysts and their enemies, all the other psychotherapists, and wish them well, but lay all your money on the neurobiologists for the decades ahead.

Pay attention to what the social scientists are saying about medicine, but don't let them argue you away from science. If anyone tells you—and many will that today's doctor is too obsessed with the disease of his patient, and not enough concerned with the patient who has the disease, don't let the moment pass without comment. Remind the critic that the disease is the main point, not the only point but the main point, of the encounter between physician and patient. Until that question is settled—and it can only be settled by science—nothing else matters, not the home environment nor the family interrelationships nor the patient's job satisfaction nor the time of day.

The first task of the doctor is to learn whether there *is* a disease, then its nature, then what to do about it. If, as turns out in about 80 per cent of encounters, there's no disease, or only a mild, self-limiting illness, there'll be other things to do for comfort and caring, but these must come later, after the disease question is settled. If I become ill, I want a doctor who can look for, and quickly recognize, the earliest signs of cancer, or heart disease, or whatever. I'll be more comforted by the presence of a physician who knows how to feel for the tip of my spleen, and what it means if it's there, than by any doctor whose education prepares him first of all to feel for my mind. My mind can wait a while, but none of the disorders which enlarge my spleen can. . . .

On the Move

The whole field of biomedical science is on the move, as never before in the long history of medicine. I don't know what will happen over the next twenty years, but my guess is that we are on the verge of discoveries that will match the best achievements in infectious disease a generation ago. As we develop new, decisive technologies that are based on a really deep understanding of disease mechanisms, my guess is that they will turn out to be relatively inexpensive compared with the kinds of measures that medicine is obliged to rely on these days for just making do. What lies ahead, if the research goes well, is a genuine high technology for medicine.

It will make an enormous difference to the practice of medicine if we can keep the basic biomedical science going and keep it coupled as congenially as possible to clinical research. We shouldn't forget how useful medicine can be when its scientific base becomes really solid and effective. The diseases that ranked as the great menaces to human health when I was a medical student on the wards of the Boston City Hospital 50 years ago were, in order of the degree of fear they caused in the public mind, tertiary syphilis of the brain (which filled more asylum beds than schizophrenia), pulmonary tuberculosis (especially in the very young and very old, for whom it was a flat death sentence), and acute rheumatic fever (far and away the commonest cause of disabling heart disease and early death). Also, of course, poliomyelitis. These four were feared by everyone, as cancer is today. Thanks to some excellent basic science, and some exceedingly classy clinical research, all four have nearly vanished as public health problems, and the vanishing involved the expenditure of pennies compared to what we would be spending if any of them were still with us. It's that level of effectiveness that I foresee for the practice of medicine.

Ranking Concerns in Health Care

The authors in this chapter debate how we should spend our health care dollars. Each author, whether intentionally or unintentionally, advocates a system of values that determines his or her priorities in health care.

This activity will give you an opportunity to discuss with classmates the values you and they consider important in health care and the values you believe are considered most important by the majority of Americans.

Part I

Step 1. Working individually, each student should rank the health care concerns listed below, assigning the number 1 to the concern he or she personally considers most important, the number 2 to the second most important concern, and so on, until all concerns have been ranked.

_____ making a profit
_____ managing hospitals efficiently
_____ providing free health care to the unemployed
_____ providing free health care to the elderly
_____ encouraging holistic treatment of patients
_____ improving health care in third world countries
_____ improving conditions in US hospitals
_____ providing better training for doctors
_____ increasing nurses' salaries
_____ acquiring more sophisticated technology
_____ improving medical diagnosis and therapy
_____ educating the public about preventive medicine

_____ finding a cure for cancer
_____ increasing Medicaid and Medicare funds
_____ curbing malpractice suits
_____ improving the physician-patient relationship
_____ finding a cure for heart disease
_____ decreasing health care costs to the average consumer

Step 2. Students should break into groups of four to six and compare their rankings with others in the group, giving reasons for their rankings.

Part 2

Step 1. Working in groups of four to six students, each group should rank the concerns listed in what the group considers the order of importance to the majority of Americans. Assign the number 1 to the concern the group believes is most important to the majority of Americans, and so on until all the concerns have been ranked.

Step 2. Each group should compare its rankings with others in a classwide discussion.

Step 3. The entire class should discuss the following questions:

1. What noticeable differences do you see between personal rankings in Part I and the perceived rankings of the majority of Americans in Part 2?
2. How would you explain these differences?
3. What conclusions do you draw about the direction health care might take if you examine (a) the majority of Americans' rankings in Part 2, and (b) your own rankings in Part 1?

Periodical Bibliography

The following list of periodical articles deals with the subject matter of this chapter.

American Medical News	"AHA Campaign Calls Attention to Plight of Medically Indigent," July 25, 1986.
Karl D. Bays	"Changing Health Care Practices," *Vital Speeches of the Day*, January 1, 1986.
Robert H. Brook and Kathleen N. Lohr	"Will We Need To Ration Effective Health Care?" *Issues in Science and Technology*, Fall 1986.
John P. Bunker	"When Doctors Disagree," *The New York Review of Books*, April 25, 1985.
Joseph A. Califano Jr.	"A Revolution Looms in American Health," *The New York Times*, March 25, 1986.
Don Colburn	"The Millions Without Health Insurance," *The Washington Post National Weekly Edition*, July 21, 1986.
Hugh Drummond	"Take Two Echocardiograms and Call Me in the Morning," *Mother Jones*, November 1986.
Erik Gunn	"Cutting Costs, Not Care," *The Washington Monthly*, June 1986.
Robert Miner	"Why Hospitals Make Mistakes," *Newsweek*, June 17, 1985.
Rita Ricardo-Campbell	"Economics and Health: The Medical Mystique," *Vital Speeches of the Day*, March 15, 1986.
George Rust	"Who Cares?: Health Care for the Poor," *Eternity*, September 1986.
Dena Seiden	"Diminishing Resources, Critical Choices," *Commonweal*, March 8, 1985.
Mark Sheldon	"Ethical Issues in the Cost-Containment of Modern Medicine," *Urban Health*, September 1984.
Society	"Compound Fracture: The American Hospital Today," July/August 1986. A series of seven articles on the American health care system.
Abigail Trafford	"Medicine's New Triumphs," *U.S. News & World Report*, November 11, 1985.

Glossary of Terms

AID *artificial insemination* in which a donor's *sperm* is used

AIH *artificial insemination* in which the husband's *sperm* is used

antigen a substance that forces the body's immune system to produce antibodies to it

artificial insemination inserting male *sperm* into a female uterus by means other than sexual intercourse in order to achieve a pregnancy

bacterium a single-celled microscopic organism that reproduces by dividing and often lives in colonies; it may exist as a free, living organism in water or soil or as a parasite in plants or animals

Barney Clark the first human recipient of an artificial heart

cadaver a dead body; specifically one intended for dissection

cell a microscopic unit of living matter which has a *nucleus*

cell fusion the combining of two or more (different kinds of) cells to become a single *cell* which has the characteristics of both

chromosomes the threadlike parts of a plant or animal cell *nucleus* which are made up of *DNA* and protein

conception the moment at which a male *sperm* and female *egg* join to create an *embryo*

conceptus the fetus

DNA deoxyribonucleic acid; the genetic material found in all living things; contains the inherited characteristics of every living organism

Draize test standard test for determining irritancy levels of cosmetics and toiletries; involves application of the chemical to be tested into the sensitive eyes of rabbits

egg the female reproductive unit; contains all the genetic material necessary, when joined with a *sperm*, to develop into a human individual

embryo in humans, the developing individual from the moment of *conception* to the end of the eighth week

embryo transfer (ET) removal of an *embryo* from an artificial environment to a uterus or from one woman's uterus to another's

gametes a mature male *sperm* or female *egg* which is capable of forming a human *embryo* if fused with a gamete of the opposite sex

gene the fundamental unit of heredity; one segment of *DNA* arranged in a specific sequence which is passed from parent to child

genetic engineering the technologies used to change the genetic makeup of a *cell* by moving or manipulating its *DNA*

genetic mother the woman whose *egg* is used to create a child, whether or not that woman carries the child

gestational mother the women who is pregnant with and delivers a child, whether or not that woman is genetically related to the child

impotent unable to engage in sexual intercourse

infertile unable to have children

***in vitro* fertilization** literally, "in glass" fertilization; fertilizing an *egg* outside the human body and in an artificial environment

IVF *in vitro* fertilization

Jarvik-7 one of the first artificial hearts; created by Robert Jarvik

LD 50 lethal dosage 50 test; aim of test is to determine the dosage level at which 50 percent of the test animals die; used to determine dangerousness of tested chemical

nucleus the dense central part of a plant or animal *cell* containing genetic material

ovum the female reproductive *egg*

plasmid hereditary material that is not part of a *chromosome*

recombinant DNA the result of combining pieces of *DNA* from different organisms

RNA ribonucleic acid; a molecule that carries the genetic message from *DNA* to a *cell*

semen fluid of the male reproductive tract which contains *sperm*

sperm the male reproductive unit; contains all the genetic material necessary, when joined with an *egg*, to develop into a human individual

surrogacy the process in which a *surrogate mother* carries a child for another woman

surrogate mother substitute; a woman who becomes pregnant in order to give the child of that pregnancy to another woman

sterile incapable of producing offspring

toxicity tests many different tests using laboratory animals, including *LD 50* and *Draize*, to determine the toxicity or irritancy of the tested chemical

vaccine a killed or partly modified *antigen* which is used to gain immunity to infectious diseases

virus an infectious organism made up of *RNA* or *DNA* in a protein coat; can only reproduce inside another *cell*

vivisection experimention that requires surgery on live animals

zygote the first *cell* formed by the union of an *egg* and *sperm*

Organizations To Contact

The editors have compiled the following list of organizations which are concerned with the issues debated in this book. All of them have publications or information available for interested readers. The descriptions are derived from materials provided by the organizations themselves.

The American Anti-Vivisectionist Society
Suite 204 Nobel Plaza
801 Old York Rd.
Jenkintown, PA 19046-1685
(215) 887-0816

Established in 1883, the Society is the oldest animal rights group in America. It opposes all live animal experimentation. Its publications include a monthly magazine and several pamphlets and position papers.

American Association for Laboratory Animal Science
210 N. Hammes Ave., Suite 205
Joliet, IL 60435
(815) 729-1161

The Association consists of persons and institutions professionally concerned with the production, use, care, and study of laboratory animals. It publishes a variety of brochures and educational materials.

American Council on Transplantation (ACT)
4701 Willard Ave., Suite 222
Chevy Chase, MD 20815
(301) 652-0994

ACT is an information referral organization for other organizations, health professionals, and individuals concerned with the donation, equitable distribution, and transplantation of organs and tissues. It publishes *Transplant Action,* a newsletter, and has a toll-free number, 1-800-ACT-GIVE.

American Fertility Society (AFS)
2131 Magnolia Ave., Suite 201
Birmingham, AL 35256
(205) 251-9764

The Society consists of gynecologists, obstetricians, urologists, reproductive endocrinologists, veterinarians, research workers, and others interested in human and animal reproduction. It seeks to extend knowledge of all aspects of fertility and problems of infertility and to provide a rostrum for the presentation of scientific studies dealing with these subjects. Publications include a monthly *Fertility and Sterility Journal* and a quarterly newsletter.

American Fund for Alternatives to Animal Research (AFAAR)
175 W. 12th St., Suite 16G
New York, NY 10011
(212) 989-8073

AFAAR sponsors research that uses non-animal experimentation in order to encourage scientists to develop alternatives to vivisection. It opposes any animal experimentation that causes pain to the animal.

American Health Foundation (AHF)
320 E. 43rd St.
New York, NY 10017
(212) 953-1900

The Foundation emphasizes four major fields in preventive medicine: research (on nutrition, environmental carcinogenesis, molecular biology, experimental pathology, and epidemiology); clinical research and service for adults and children; public health action; and health economics research. It publishes *Preventive Medicine* quarterly and was formerly called the Environmental Health Foundation.

American Medical Association (AMA)
535 N. Dearborn St.
Chicago, IL 60610
(312) 645-5000

The AMA is a professional association for physicians. Publications include *American Medical News* and *Journal of the American Medical Association*, both weeklies.

Association for Gnotobiotics
Department of Dermatology
Roswell Park Institute
666 Elm St.
Buffalo, NY 14263

The Association works to stimulate research in the field of applied gnotobiotics, or the science of maintaining a controlled environment. It provides information for scientists who use live animals on how to raise these animals in a controlled environment for research. Its publications include position papers and a newsletter.

Association of Biotechnology Companies (ABC)
Dr. Bruce F. Mackler
General Council
1220 L St. NW, Suite 615
Washington, DC 20005
(202) 842-2229

ABC provides information on biotechnology issues pertaining to regulations, patents, and finance. The Association's publications include *ABC Alerts, Dialog* newsletter, and monthly columns in biotechnology journals.

Beauty Without Cruelty
175 W. 12th St.
New York, NY 10011
(212) 989-8073

Beauty Without Cruelty seeks to inform the public about the massive suffering of many kinds of animals in the fashion and cosmetics industries. It provides information about substitute fashions and cosmetics which have not involved death, confinement, or suffering of any animal. It publishes a newsletter and position statements.

Biomedical Research Defense Fund (BRDF)
819 E. Fayette St., Suite 584
Baltimore, MD 21202

BRDF provides funds to defend scientists and research organizations whose rights to carry out biomedical animal research are being threatened or impaired. It provides the public with information on biomedical animal research and its importance to medical advancement.

Center for Medical Consumers and Health Care Information (CMC)
237 Thompson St.
New York, NY 10012
(212) 674-7105

The Center encourages people to make a critical evaluation of all information received from health professions; to use medical services more selectively; to understand the limitations of modern medicine; and to understand that lifestyle choices such as smoking, exercise habits, and nutritional practices have a greater effect on health than does access to medical care. CMC conducts research and publishes its results.

Committee for Responsible Genetics (CRG)
186-A South St.
Boston, MA 02111
(617) 423-0560

CRG consists of scientists, health and medical professionals, trade unionists, feminists, and peace activists. The organization monitors and analyzes the biotechnology industry and discusses the social implications of biotechnological developments. Areas of interest include military uses of biological research and the social implications of new reproductive technologies such as prenatal testing. It maintains a resource center and publishes *Gene Watch*, a bimonthly bulletin.

Fertility Research Foundation (FRF)
1430 2nd Ave., Suite 103
New York, NY 10021
(212) 744-5500

The Foundation specializes in human reproduction. It provides therapeutic, diagnostic, and consultation service for childless couples; conducts infertility surveys; maintains research projects; and conducts programs for practicing physicians, residents, and medical students on how to educate the public. It publishes the bimonthly *Fertility Review* and the quarterly *Infertility.*

Foundation for Biomedical Research
818 Connecticut Ave. NW, Suite 303
Washington, DC 20006
(202) 457-0654

The Foundation consists of individuals and organizations supporting humane animal research. It provides public information and education on what the foundation sees as the necessity and important role of laboratory animals in biomedical research and testing. Publications include a newsletter and position papers.

The Hastings Center
360 Broadway
Hastings-on-Hudson, NY 10706
(914) 478-0500

Since its founding in 1969, The Hastings Center has played a central role in raising issues as a response to advances in medicine, the biological sciences, and the social and behavioral sciences. In examining the wide range of moral, social, and legal questions, the Center had established three goals: advancement of research on ethical issues, stimulation of universities and professional schools to support the teaching of ethics, and public education. It publishes *The Hastings Center Report.*

Institute of Laboratory Animal Resources
National Research Council
2102 Constitution Ave. NW

Washington, DC 20418
(202) 334-2590

The Institute maintains an information center and answers inquiries concerning animal models for biomedical research. Its committees develop guidelines on breeding and human care and use of laboratory animals. It publishes a quarterly newsletter.

International Society for Animal Rights, Inc.
421 S. State St.
Clarks Summit, PA 18411
(717) 586-2200

The Society opposes the use of animals in biomedical and related research. It publishes a bimonthly newsletter, alerts on pending legislation, books, pamphlets, monographs, films, and videos.

Living Bank (LB)
P.O. Box 6725
Houston, TX 77265
1-800-528-2971

The Living Bank is a national registry and referral service created to help those persons who, upon death, wish to donate organs and/or tissues for the purpose of transplantation, therapy, or medical research. The Bank maintains a lending library of films for the public, hospitals, and police departments. It also provides educational materials for the public on organ donation and publishes *The Bank Account*, a quarterly newsletter.

National Association for Biomedical Research
818 Connecticut Ave. NW, Suite 303
Washington, DC 20006
(202) 857-0540

The Association is comprised of various professionals from the biomedical field who monitor, and when appropriate, attempt to influence legislation and regulations on behalf of members who are dependent on animals for biomedical research and testing. It publishes numerous materials.

National Committee for Quality Health Care (NCQHC)
1730 Rhode Island Ave. NW, Suite 803
Washington, DC 20036
(202) 861-0882

NCQHC is a coalition of health care professionals and organizations principally involved in the health care industry. It includes hospitals, physicians, health maintenance organizations, nursing homes, manufacturers of health care equipment, investment bankers, architects, contractors, and accountants. The Committee believes that "government intervention is not the answer." It publishes *Capital Outlook* monthly and provides papers and pamphlets.

People for the Ethical Treatment of Animals (PETA)
P.O. Box 42516
Washington, DC 20015
(202) 726-0516

PETA is one of the largest animal rights organizations and opposes all live animal experimentation. It publishes numerous books, pamphlets, and brochures.

Psychologists for the Ethical Treatment of Animals (PsyEta)
c/o Psychology Department
Bates College
Lewiston, ME 04240
(207) 926-4817

PsyEta is a group of psychologists who share a common concern that psychology reexamine its treatment of research animals. The group represents a variety of opinions ranging from the retention of animal research to its abolition. It publishes numerous pamphlets and position papers.

Rural Advancement Fund International (RAFI)
P.O. Box 1029
Pittsboro, NC 27312
(919) 542-5292

RAFI is a conservation organization concerned about the loss of genetic diversity in plants and animals. It publishes the quarterly *RAFI Report.*

Scientists Center for Animal Welfare
4905 St. Elmo
Bethesda, MD 20814
(301) 654-6390

The Center is an organization of scientists who study or are concerned about their responsibilities to laboratory animals. The scientists believe a humane concern for animals should be incorporated into the conduct of science. The organization publishes a book and position papers.

Society for Animal Protective Legislation
P.O. Box 3719
Washington, DC 20007
(202) 337-2332

The Society works for and has succeeded in having bills passed to insure animal rights. It lobbies for humane treatment of experimental animals, the abolition of steel traps, stronger endangered species laws, and other efforts. Publications include several brochures, informational packets, and position papers.

Student Action Corps for Animals
P.O. Box 15588
Washington, DC 20003-0588
(202) 543-8983

This student group opposes the use of live-animal dissection in high schools. Believing students have the right to not participate in dissection in schools, the group publishes newsletters and articles advocating this view.

Trans-Species Unlimited
P.O. Box 1553
Williamsport, PA 17703-1553
(717) 332-3252

This all-volunteer organization is committed to total elimination of animal abuse and exploitation. The group encourages the use of cruelty-free cosmetics and fashions, and its actions include raids and sit-ins to stop illegal vivisection. It publishes brochures and position papers.

Bibliography of Books

Henry Aaron and
William B. Schwartz

The Painful Prescription: Rationing Hospital Care. Washington, DC: The Brookings Institution, 1984.

Lori B. Andrews

New Conceptions. New York: St. Martin's Press, 1984.

Animal Welfare
Institute

Beyond the Laboratory Door. Washington, DC: The Animal Welfare Institute, 1985.

Rita Arditti, Renate
Duelli Klein, and
Shelley Minden, eds.

Test-Tube Women: What Future for Motherhood? Boston: Pandora Press, 1984.

T. Beauchamp and
L. Walters, eds.

Contemporary Issues in Bioethics, 2nd Edition. Belmont, CA: Wadsworth, 1982.

Robert Boakes

From Darwin to Behaviorism: Psychology and the Minds of Animals. Cambridge, MA: Cambridge University Press, 1984.

Joseph A. Califano Jr.

America's Health Care Revolution. New York: Random House, 1986.

Gena Corea

The Mother Machine: Reproductive Technologies from Artificial Insemination to Artificial Wombs. New York: Harper & Row, 1985.

Robert M. Cunningham
Jr.

The Healing Mission and the Business Ethic. Chicago: Pluribus Press, 1982.

Patricia Curtis

Animal Rights. New York: Four Winds Press, 1980.

Norman Daniels

Just Health Care. New York: Cambridge University Press, 1985.

Bernard D. Davis

Storm Over Biology. Buffalo, NY: Prometheus Books, 1986.

W. Jean Dodds and
F. Barbara Orlans, eds.

Scientific Perspectives on Animal Welfare. Orlando, FL: Academic Press, 1986.

Harry F. Dowling

Fighting Infection: Conquests of the Twentieth Century. Cambridge, MA: Harvard University Press, 1977.

Jack Doyle

Altered Harvest. New York: The Viking Press, 1985.

H. Tristram
Engelhardt Jr.

The Foundations of Bioethics. New York: Oxford University Press, 1986.

Joseph Fletcher

Humanhood: Essays in Biomedical Ethics. Buffalo, NY: Prometheus Books, 1979.

Michael Allen Fox

The Case for Animal Experimentation. Los Angeles: University of California Press, 1986.

R.G. Frey

Interests and Rights: The Case Against Animals. Oxford: Clarendon Press, 1980.

Lawrence Galton

Medical Advances. Harmondsworth, Middlesex, England: Penguin Books, 1979.

Samuel Gorovitz	*Doctors' Dilemmas: Moral Conflict and Medical Care.* New York: MacMillan Publishing Co., Inc., 1982.
Bradford H. Gray, ed.	*The New Health Care for Profit: Doctors and Hospitals in a Competitive Environment.* Washington, DC: National Academy Press, 1983.
Alan Herscovivi	*Second Nature:* The Animal Rights Controversy. Toronto: CBC Enterprises, 1985.
David Hilfiker	*Healing the Wounds: A Physician Looks at His Work.* New York: Pantheon, 1985.
D. Gareth Jones	*Brave New People.* Grand Rapids, MI: William B. Eerdmans, 1984.
Noel Keane and Denis Breo	*The Surrogate Mother.* New York: Everest House, 1981.
Daniel J. Kevles	*In the Name of Eugenics: Genetics and the Uses of Human Heredity.* New York: Alfred A. Knopf, 1985.
Sheldon J. Krimsky	*Genetic Alchemy: The Social History of the Recombinant DNA Controversy.* Cambridge, MA: MIT Press, 1982.
Marc Lappé	*Broken Code: The Exploitation of DNA.* San Francisco: Sierra Club Books, 1984.
Gerald Leinwand	*Transplants: Today's Medical Miracles.* New York: Franklin Watts, 1985.
Michael Lockwood	*Moral Dilemmas in Modern Medicine.* New York: Oxford University Press, 1986.
James B. Maas, ed.	*Readings in Psychology Today.* New York: Random House, 1979.
James B. Nelson and Jo Anne Smith Rohricht	*Human Medicine: Ethical Perspectives on Today's Medical Issues.* Minneapolis: Augsburg Publishing House, 1984.
J. Robert Nelson	*Human Life: A Biblical Perspective for Bioethics.* Philadelphia: Fortress Press, 1984.
Karen O'Connor	*Sharing the Kingdom: Animals and Their Rights.* New York: Dodd, Mead & Company, 1984.
Sandra Panem, ed.	*Biotechnology: Implications for Public Policy.* Washington, DC: The Brookings Institution, 1985.
President's Commission for the Study of Ethical Problems in Medicine and Biomedical and Behavioral Research	*Splicing Life: The Social and Ethical Issues of Genetic Engineering with Human Beings.* Washington, DC: US Government Printing Office, 1982.
Phychologists for the Ethical Treatment of Animals	*Position Papers by the Dozen.* Available for $2 from PsyEta, c/o Psychology Department, Bates College, Lewiston, ME, 14240.
Tom Regan	*Animal Sacrifices: Religious Perspectives on the Use of Animals in Science.* Philadelphia: Temple University Press, 1986.
Tom Regan	*The Case for Animal Rights.* Berkeley, CA: University of California Press, 1983.

211

Jeremy Rifkin	*Algeny*. New York: The Viking Press, 1983.
Andrew Rowan	*Of Mice, Models and Men: A Critical Evaluation of Animal Research*. Albany, NY: State University of New York Press, 1984.
Hans Ruesch	*Slaughter of the Innocent*. New York: Bantam Books, 1978.
Russell Scott	*The Body as Property*. London: Allen Lane, 1981.
Margery W. Shaw, ed.	*After Barney Clark: Reflections on the Utah Artificial Heart Program*. Austin, TX: University of Texas Press, 1984.
Peter Singer	*Animal Liberation: A New Ethics for Our Treatment of Animals*. New York: Avon Books, 1975.
Peter Singer, ed.	*In Defense of Animals*. New York: Basil Blackwell, 1985.
Peter Singer and Deane Wells	*Making Babies: The New Science and Ethics of Conception*. New York: Charles Scribner's Sons, 1984.
R. Snowden and G.D. Mitchell	*The Artificial Family*. London: Allen and Unwin, 1981.
Frank Stilley	*The $100,000 Rat and Other Animal Heroes for Humane Health*. New York: G.P. Putnam's, 1975.
Mary Warnock	*A Question of Life*. Oxford: Basil Blackwell, 1985.
James D. Watson and Jon Tooze	*The DNA Story: A Documentary History of Gene Cloning*. San Francisco: Freeman, 1981.
Edward Yoxen	*The Gene Business: Who Should Control Biotechnology?* New York: Harper & Row, 1983.

Index

medicine, improvement of
  by holistic techniques, 190-193
  by scientific research, 196-199
Meissner, Joseph, 177
Mendel, Gregor, 17
Mendelsohn, Everett, 59, 60
Meyer, Charles, 95
Moore, John, 74, 75, 77
Morreim, E. Haavi, 183
Muggeridge, Malcolm, 69
Murray, Thomas H., 73

National Organ Transplantation Act,
  80-81
Nelson, James B., 75
Ness, Richard, 55

organ transplants
  and curing diseases, 197
  availability of, 68, 70-71, 186
  costs of, 66-67
  destroy human values, 69-72
  economic reasons against, 86
  improved success rate in, 68
  laws concerning, 75, 76, 77, 79,
    80-81
  need for, 65-68
  statistics on, 66, 80
  types of, 66-68
  see also artificial heart
organs
  purchase of
    Congressional ban on, 76, 79, 81
    is practical, 78-81
    is unethical, 73-77
  views of
    as gift, 76-77
    is unrealistic, 79
    as property, 75-76, 81
Otteson, Gary, 159
Ozar, David T., 121

Peck, Keenan, 25, 34
Pillar, Charles, 59
poor, health care for, see health care
Pope Pius XII, 117
pseudorabies
  livestock vaccine for, 38, 39, 52,
    56-57

quality of life
  formula for determining, 181
  is discriminatory, 182

Rabin, Robert, 57
Ramsey, Paul, 97
Rassaby, Alan A., 108
Regan, Tom, 149

reproductive technology
  and attitudes toward infertility, 101
  artificial insemination by donor
    and adoption, 100, 102, 106
    keeping records of, 98, 107
    laws concerning, 98, 104
    reasons against, 97, 100-101
    reasons for, 104
    risks of, 98, 105, 106-107
    should be restricted, 95-102
      con, 103-107
  frozen embryos
    and abortion issue, 124-125,
      133-134
    cost of, 128-129
    destruction of
      is acceptable, 130-136
      is wrong, 121-129
    morality of, 123-124, 129, 131,
      135-136
    Rios case, 122
  in vitro fertilization, 96-97, 99, 101,
    105
    and surrogate motherhood, 118
    definition of, 105
  semen donors' role in, 98, 104
    screening of, 97-98
  surrogate motherhood
    and adoption, 109, 111, 112
    and adultery, 109, 110
    custody disputes in, 113-114,
      118-120
    devalues children, 116, 117, 120
      fallacy of, 111
    should be allowed, 108-114
    should not be allowed, 115-120
Ricardo-Campbell, Rita, 171
Rifkin, Jeremy, 23, 52
Roe v. Wade, 124-125
Rohricht, Jo Anne Smith, 75

Schwartz, Harry, 82
science
  and profit, 76, 77
  and social sciences, 198
  can improve medical care, 196-199
    history of, 199
    limits to, 192-193
  impact of changes in, 20, 21
  must be limited, 190-191
Seavey, David, 53
Simmons, Paul D., 110
Singer, Peter, 107, 130
Snyder, Paul, 191
Sparks, Samantha, 57
Stuller, Jay, 20
Surrogate Parenting Associates v.
  Kentucky, 116

215